Evaluation and Management of Obstructive Sleep Apnea

Guest Editor

SCOTT B. BOYD, DDS, PhD

ORAL AND MAXILLOFACIAL SURGERY CLINICS OF NORTH AMERICA

www.oralmaxsurgery.theclinics.com

Consulting Editor

RICHARD H. HAUG, DDS

November 2009 • Volume 21 • Number 4

SAUNDERS an imprint of ELSEVIER, Inc.

W.B. SAUNDERS COMPANY
A Division of Elsevier Inc.

1600 John F. Kennedy Blvd. • Suite 1800 • Philadelphia, PA 19103-2899

www.oralmaxsurgery.theclinics.com

ORAL AND MAXILLOFACIAL SURGERY CLINICS OF NORTH AMERICA Volume 21, Number 4
November 2009 ISSN 1042-3699, ISBN-13: 978-1-4377-1251-3, ISBN-10: 1-4377-1251-7

Editor: John Vassallo; j.vassallo@elsevier.com

Oral and Maxillofacial Surgery Clinics of North America (ISSN 1042-3699) is published quarterly by Elsevier Inc., 360 Park Avenue South, New York, NY 10010-1710. Months of issue are February, May, August, and November. Business and Editorial Offices: 1600 John F. Kennedy Blvd., Suite 1800, Philadelphia, PA 19103-2899. Periodicals postage paid at New York, NY and additional mailing offices. Subscription prices are $271.00 per year for US individuals, $401.00 per year for US institutions, $125.00 per year for US students and residents, $313.00 per year for Canadian individuals, $478.00 per year for Canadian institutions, $362.00 per year for international individuals, $478.00 per year for international institutions and $170.00 per year for Canadian and foreign students/residents. To receive student/resident rate, orders must be accompanied by name or affiliated institution, date of term, and the *signature* of program/residency coordinator on institution letterhead. Orders will be billed at individual rate until proof of status is received. Foreign air speed delivery is included in all *Clinics* subscription prices. All prices are subject to change without notice. **POSTMASTER:** Send address changes to *Oral and Maxillofacial Surgery Clinics of North America,* Elsevier Periodicals Customer Service, 11830 Westline Industrial Drive, St. Louis, MO 63146. Tel: 1-800-654-2452 (U.S. and Canada); 314-453-7041 (outside U.S. and Canada). Fax: 314-523-5170. E-mail: journalscustomerservice-usa@elsevier.com (for print support); journalsonlinesupport-usa@elsevier.com (for online support).

Reprints. For copies of 100 or more, of articles in this publication, please contact the Commercial Reprints Department, Elsevier Inc., 360 Park Avenue South, New York, NY 10010-1710. Tel.: 212-633-3812; Fax: 212-462-1935; Email: reprints@elsevier.com.

Oral and Maxillofacial Surgery Clinics of North America is covered in MEDLINE/PubMed (*Index Medicus*).

Printed and bound by CPI Group (UK) Ltd, Croydon, CR0 4YY

Transferred to Digital Print 2011

Contributors

CONSULTING EDITOR

RICHARD H. HAUG, DDS
Carolinas Center for Oral Health
Charlotte, North Carolina

GUEST EDITOR

SCOTT B. BOYD, DDS, PhD
Research Professor, Vanderbilt School
of Medicine, Nashville, Tennessee

AUTHORS

FERNANDA R. ALMEIDA, DDS, MSc, PhD
Clinical Assistant Professor, Department of
Oral Biological and Medical Sciences, The
University of British Columbia, Vancouver,
British Columbia, Canada

CARL BOUCHARD, DMD, MSc, FRCD (C)
AO/ASIF/MGH Fellow in Pediatric Oral and
Maxillofacial Surgery and Instructor in Oral and
Maxillofacial Surgery, Department of Oral and
Maxillofacial Surgery, Massachusetts General
Hospital, Harvard School of Dental Medicine,
Boston, Massachusetts

SCOTT B. BOYD, DDS, PhD
Research Professor, Vanderbilt School
of Medicine, Nashville, Tennessee

LEONARD B. KABAN, DMD, MD
Walter C. Guralnick Professor and Chairman,
Department of Oral and Maxillofacial Surgery,
Massachusetts General Hospital, Harvard
School of Dental Medicine, Boston,
Massachusetts

N. RAY LEE, DDS
Assistant Clinical Professor, Department of
Oral and Maxillofacial Surgery, Medical
College of Virginia, Virginia Commonwealth
University, Richmond, Virginia; Private
Practice, Oyster Point Oral and Facial Surgery,
Newport News, Virginia

KASEY K. LI, MD, DDS, FACS
Adjunct Clinical Associate Professor,
Surgical Director, Multi-disciplinary Treatment
Team, Stanford Sleep Disorders Clinic and
Research Center, Stanford, California

**ALAN A. LOWE, DMD, DipOrtho, PhD,
FRCD (C), FCDS (BC)**
Professor and Chair, Division of Orthodontics,
Department of Oral Health Sciences, The
University of British Columbia, Vancouver,
British Columbia, Canada

FARIDEH MADANI, DMD
Clinical Professor of Oral Medicine, School of
Dental Medicine, University of Pennsylvania,
Philadelphia, Pennsylvania

MANSOOR MADANI, DMD, MD
Chairman, Department of Oral and
Maxillofacial Surgery, Capital Health, Trenton,
New Jersey; Associate Professor, Oral &
Maxillofacial Surgery, Temple University,
Philadelphia, Pennsylvania; Director, Center for
Corrective Jaw Surgery, Bala Cynwyd,
Pennsylvania

SAMUEL A. MICKELSON, MD, FACS, ABSM
Advanced Ear Nose & Throat Associates PC,
Atlanta, Georgia; Director, The Atlanta Snoring
and Sleep Disorders Institute, Atlanta,
Georgia

PETER D. O'CONNOR, MD, OD
Sleep Medicine Fellow, Department of
Otolaryngology and Communication Sciences,
Medical College of Wisconsin, Milwaukee,
Wisconsin

AMY SAWYER, PhD, RN
Postdoctoral Fellow, Biobehavioral and
Health Sciences Division, University of
Pennsylvania School of Nursing,
Philadelphia, Pennsylvania

SOMSAK SITTITAVORNWONG, DDS, MS
UAB Oral and Maxillofacial Surgery, University
of Alabama Birmingham, Birmingham,
Alabama

MARIA J. TROULIS, DDS, MSc
Associate Professor of Oral and Maxillofacial
Surgery, and Residency Program; Director,
Department of Oral and Maxillofacial Surgery,

Massachusetts General Hospital, Harvard
School of Dental Medicine, Boston,
Massachusetts

PETER D. WAITE, DDS, MD, MPH
UAB Oral and Maxillofacial Surgery, University
of Alabama Birmingham, Birmingham,
Alabama

TERRI E. WEAVER, PhD, RN, FAAN
Professor and Chair, Biobehavioral and
Health Sciences Division, University of
Pennsylvania School of Nursing,
Philadelphia, Pennsylvania

B. TUCKER WOODSON, MD
Professor and Chief, Division of Sleep
Medicine, Department of Otolaryngology
and Communication Sciences, Medical
College of Wisconsin, Milwaukee,
Wisconsin

Contents

The normal cycle of respiration includes a unique balancing force between many upper airway structures that control its dilation and closure. Alteration of this delicate equilibrium, possibly by an increased airflow resistance, can cause various degrees of obstructive sleep apnea (OSA). OSA is now recognized as a major illness, an important cause of medical morbidity and mortality affecting millions of people worldwide, and a major predisposing factor for several systemic conditions, such as hypertension, cardiovascular disease, stroke, diabetes, and even sexual dysfunction. Initial evaluation for possible OSA may be done by dental professionals who can provide guidance for its comprehensive evaluation and management. Because of the complexity of the disease, factors contributing to its development must be identified. Some factors caused by the patient's anatomic structures are slightly easier to rectify, whereas others may relate to the patient's age, sex, habits, or associated illnesses, including obesity. In this article, various epidemiologic, pathophysiologic, and clinical features of OSA are discussed.

This article provides a practical strategy for the systematic evaluation of the obstructive sleep apnea patient. The management of snoring is also discussed. The presented strategy is based upon review of the current literature, the principles set forth in the American Academy of Sleep Medicine clinical guideline publication, and the author's personal experience.

Obstructive sleep apnea syndrome is an increasingly common disorder, but the etiology and site of obstruction often remain unknown. The obstruction seldom is imaged or identified. All surgical procedures must be directed toward the anatomic site of obstruction. Currently, it is very difficult to identify the site of obstruction in the awake, nonsupine patient. Therefore, better diagnostic methods must be developed to help direct treatment options and improve surgical outcomes. This article will help surgeons identify possible sites of obstruction and direct surgical intervention.

Obstructive sleep apnea (OSA) is a common problem, with 9% to 28% of women and 24% to 26% of males having apneic events at a treatable level, making this syndrome a serious public health issue. This article describes the outcomes associated with continuous positive airway pressure treatment, significance of the issue of poor adherence in OSA, discusses evidence regarding the optimal duration of nightly use, describes the nature and predictors of nonadherence, and reviews interventions that have been tested to increase nightly use and suggests management strategies.

Principles of Oral Appliance Therapy for the Management of Snoring and Sleep Disordered Breathing

Fernanda R. Almeida and Alan A. Lowe

Oral appliance (OA) therapy for snoring, obstructive sleep apnea, or both is simple, reversible, quiet, and cost-effective and may be indicated in patients who are unable to tolerate nasal continuous positive airway pressure (nCPAP) or are poor surgical risks. OAs are effective in varying degrees and seem to work because of an increase in airway space, the provision of a stable anterior position of the mandible, advancement of the tongue or soft palate, and possibly a change in genioglossus muscle activity. This article provides a detailed clinical protocol and titration sequence for OAs, because this clinical procedure is often not well understood by practitioners new to the field. Prediction of treatment success is addressed, OA treatment is compared with surgery and nCPAP, OA compliance is described, and the possible adverse effects associated with this type of therapy are discussed.

Sleep Apnea Surgery: Putting It All Together

Kasey K. Li

Since the first description of uvulopalatopharyngoplasty (UPPP) in 1972, the surgical management of obstructive sleep apnea syndrome (OSA) has become increasingly popular. This popularity is caused by several reasons. The psychomotor sequelae of OSA, such as excessive daytime sleepiness, daytime fatigue, and poor sleep quality caused by sleep fragmentation, have major deleterious impact on patients' well being, which behooves them to seek treatment. The risk of hypertension, heart attack, and stroke also prompts patients to seek treatment. Further, despite the potential success of nasal continuous positive airway pressure (CPAP), patients' compliance represents a clear problem, thus causing patients to seek treatment alternatives, namely surgery. All surgeons treating patients who have OSA must realize that the management of OSA crosses specialty lines and no single specialty can adequately take care of patients alone.

Anesthetic and Postoperative Management of the Obstructive Sleep Apnea Patient

Samuel A. Mickelson

Sleep apnea patients pose a challenge for surgeons, anesthesiologists, and surgical facilities as there is increased risk for anesthetic and postoperative complications. Precautions before and after surgery minimize these risks. Screening for sleep apnea should be done for all surgical patients. Safe perioperative management requires judicious use of narcotics and sedating medications, reducing upper airway edema, prevention of aspiration and deep vein thrombosis, blood pressure control, use of positive airway pressure, and proper postoperative monitoring. Although the literature lacks specific recommendations, the guidelines presented in this article are based on more than 20 years of experience and supported by peer-reviewed medical literature.

Reconstruction of Airway Soft Tissues in Obstructive Sleep Apnea

B. Tucker Woodson and Peter D. O'Connor

Surgery for obstructive sleep apnea is multimodal. Procedures and aims of treatment vary. Surgery, medical devices, and medical therapy each may contribute to individualized patient care. There is no single procedure or intervention that "cures" upper airway obstruction. Treatment varies as the disease varies. In addition, surgical treatment varies because the level of obstruction and influence on air flow occurs at multiple levels and from many structures. This article is not intended as a critical assessment of surgical outcomes but rather focuses on airway structures and the nature of the procedures applied to influence them.

Obstructive sleep apnea (OSA) is a common primary sleep disorder. It is characterized by repetitive partial or complete upper airway collapse during sleep. Maxillomandibular advancement (MMA) is an orthognathic surgical procedure that has been used to manage OSA. The main objective of this article is to provide practical guidelines for evaluating and managing OSA patients by MMA. The presentation will focus on MMA for adults, as this is the most common and clinically effective application of MMA to treat OSA.

Distraction osteogenesis to expand the facial skeleton is an alternative to standard orthognathic surgery for selected patients with obstructive sleep apnea. For children with congenital micrognathia or midface hypoplasia, distraction osteogenesis allows large advancements without the need for bone grafting and with less risk of relapse. For later-onset obstructive sleep apnea, distraction osteogenesis may represent an alternative when acute bone movement is expected to be difficult (scarring from previous surgery or radiation therapy) or when the risk for inferior alveolar nerve damage is unacceptable (patients older than 40 years).

Oral and Maxillofacial Surgery Clinics of North America

Preface

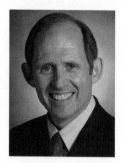

Scott B. Boyd, DDS, PhD
Guest Editor

Sleep-related problems affect over 50 million Americans of all ages and are therefore a significant public health concern. One of the most common sleep disorders is obstructive sleep apnea (OSA), which is characterized by repetitive complete or partial collapse of the upper airway during sleep. The ensuing reduction in airflow leads to hypoxia and subsequent arousals from sleep, producing sleep deprivation. Major risk factors for OSA include being male, obese, and over 40 years of age, but anyone can be affected, even children. The effect that OSA has on general health and quality of life has been well documented. Untreated OSA is associated with a significant number of medical conditions, including hypertension, myocardial infarction, and stroke. Additionally, sleep deprivation may lead to impaired cognitive function, which can hurt job performance and lead to more motor vehicle crashes. OSA is considered to be a chronic disorder that often requires lifelong management. Unfortunately, the majority of individuals with OSA are undiagnosed and therefore remain untreated.

Because of the complexity of the disease and the associated medical conditions, a broad spectrum of clinicians play important roles in the treatment of OSA. These clinicians include sleep medicine specialists, surgeons, dentists, primary care physicians, and pediatricians. Therefore, the evaluation and management of OSA are best performed using a multidisciplinary team approach. Oral and maxillofacial surgeons are integral members of the team, particularly in regard to surgical management of both adults and children with OSA.

The overarching goal of this issue is to provide contemporary guidelines for the evaluation and management of OSA in this rapidly evolving area of clinical practice. This publication is organized in an integrated fashion, so the articles are presented in a manner that generally parallels the sequence of patient care. Experts from a variety of specialties were recruited to contribute articles, thereby facilitating comprehensive coverage of the subject. Each author has done an admirable job of covering his or her topic using a blend of evidence-based review of the literature and personal experience.

I am deeply indebted and grateful to each of the authors, who have devoted their time and shared their knowledge and clinical expertise. Their high-quality articles should stand as an important resource for oral and maxillofacial surgeons providing care for patients with OSA. Additionally, this issue could not have been created without the tremendous support and incredible patience of John Vassallo, editor of the *Oral and Maxillofacial Surgery Clinics of North America*, and his production staff.

Finally, I have been incredibly fortunate to be surrounded by amazing individuals in both my professional and personal life. I was truly privileged to be trained by many of the giants of our specialty, including (in alphabetical order): William H. Bell, Bruce N. Epker, Rick A. Finn, Douglas P. Sinn, and Robert V. Walker. Each of them were incredible role models and, by example, demonstrated how to achieve excellence in patient care and advance our specialty through high-quality

Oral Maxillofacial Surg Clin N Am 21 (2009) ix–x
doi:10.1016/j.coms.2009.10.001

oralmaxsurgery.theclinics.com

resident training and production of high-impact clinical research. Without their support and mentorship, I could not have pursued a career in academic oral and maxillofacial surgery. On a personal note, I acknowledge and am forever indebted to my wife, Catherine, and to my children, Bradley, David, Lindsay, and Emily, for their love and unfailing support.

Scott B. Boyd, DDS, PhD
Vanderbilt School of Medicine
CCC 3322 MCN 2103
1161 21st Avenue South
Nashville, TN 37232-2103, USA

E-mail address:
scott.boyd@vanderbilt.edu

Epidemiology, Pathophysiology, and Clinical Features of Obstructive Sleep Apnea

Mansoor Madani, DMD, MD[a,b,c],*, Farideh Madani, DMD[d]

KEYWORDS
- Sleep apnea • Snoring • Upper airway • Obesity

CLINICAL SYMPTOMS

It is well known that snoring is one of the primary symptoms of obstructive sleep apnea (OSA). Some snorers are not aware of their problem, so an interview with the spouse or bed partner is essential.[1–9] A pattern of intermittent loud snoring interspersed with periods of silence lasting more than 10 seconds suggests the presence of OSA. Another prominent symptom is excessive daytime sleepiness. This subjective complaint can be assessed objectively with multiple sleep latency tests or with subjective questionnaires, such as the Epworth Sleepiness Scale. Other symptoms may include nocturnal arousals, nocturnal diaphoresis, abnormal motor activity during sleep, enuresis, gastroesophageal reflex, morning headaches, chest pain, diminished libido, impotence, loss of memory and concentration, and depression. Neck circumference and the degree of obesity are important predictors of sleep apnea.[10–12] Neck circumference was shown to be a more useful predictor of OSA than the presence of obesity.

PHYSIOLOGIC MECHANISMS UNDERLYING EPIDEMIOLOGIC RISK FACTORS

Although obesity is considered as the key predisposing and definitive risk factor of OSA, one must understand that there are numerous other issues that contribute to this illness. They include the patient's gender, race, family history and hereditary background, various anatomic, physiologic, and hormonal factors, and social and behavioral issues.[13–18] Anatomic factors alone could be structural abnormalities in the hard and soft tissues of maxillofacial structures leading to an increased anatomic compromise, increased pharyngeal dilator muscle dysfunction, lowered arousal threshold, increased instability of ventilatory control, or reduced lung volume tethering. Despite significant advancements in the understanding of the mechanism and the consequences of OSA, most patients affected with this problem are undiagnosed. Most patients arrive in the author's centers complaining of snoring, daytime sleepiness, poor sleep patterns, or complaints from their bed partners. Unlike other medical

[a] Department of Oral and Maxillofacial Surgery, Capital Health, Trenton, NJ 08638, USA
[b] Department of Oral & Maxillofacial Surgery, Temple University Hospital, 3401 N. Broad Street, Philadelphia, PA 19140, USA
[c] Center for Corrective Jaw Surgery, 15 North Presidential Boulevard, Suite 301, Bala Cynwyd, PA 19004, USA
[d] Department of Oral Medicine, The Robert Schattner Center, University of Pennsylvania School of Dental Medicine, 240 South 40th Street, Philadelphia, PA 19104-6030, USA
* Corresponding author. Center for Corrective Jaw Surgery, 15 North Presidential Boulevard, Suite 301, Bala Cynwyd, PA 19004.
E-mail address: drmmadani@gmail.com (M. Madani).

Oral Maxillofacial Surg Clin N Am 21 (2009) 369–375
doi:10.1016/j.coms.2009.09.003

disorders that are easily recognizable by patients, this illness only affects them in sleep and patients are unaware of its presence.

OSA occurs in approximately 4% to 9% of middle-aged men and in 1% to 2% of middle-aged women. The prevalence of OSA is highest among men aged 40 to 65 years. It seems to decrease after age 65, although more than 25% of the population older than 65 years have more than 5 apnea episodes per hour of sleep.

Although OSA mainly affects adults, its presence in children should not be ignored. The prevalence in children aged 2 to 8 years is only 2%, but the consequences may include hypertension, nocturnal enuresis, growth retardation, cognitive impairment, and hyperactivity.

Anatomic Factors

It is commonly assumed that obesity with enlargement of the soft tissue structures in the upper airway is the predominant mechanism of OSA. It is also a known fact that upper airway abnormalities play an important role in increasing its propensity to collapse during sleep, even if the individual is not obese. The exact location of collapse varies in different individuals, the main reason for failure of various surgical procedures or devices fabricated to treat OSA (**Fig. 1**). Comprehensive clinical examination and radiographic analyses using panoramic and cephalometric studies, computerized tomography, and magnetic resonance imaging have demonstrated that there are many skeletal and soft-tissue structural differences between individuals with and without OSA during wakefulness. Although the retropositioning of the tongue is one of the most common features of patients with OSA, the dimension of pharyngeal lumen and the elongation of the uvula and soft palatal draping also seem to play important roles (**Fig. 2**). Other features particularly in nonobese patients may include maxilla-mandibular retrognathism, receded chin, inferiorly positioned hyoid bone, tonsillar hypertrophy, deviated septum, nasal polyp, and enlarged nasal turbinates. The fatty deposits in the neck and the pharyngeal airway space and the thickness of pharyngeal muscles are definitely other factors that decrease posterior airway space, narrow upper airway dimensions, and promote apnea and hypopnea during sleep. One should distinguish the causes of snoring and OSA that may be common but are limited to less anatomic factors. Snoring intensity could be significantly

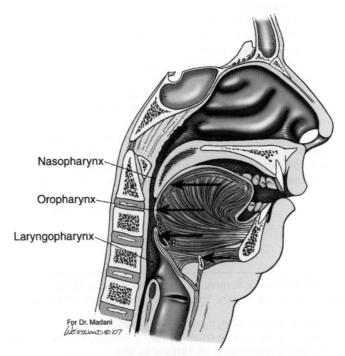

Nasopharynx

Oropharynx

Laryngopharynx

For Dr. Madani
WESTWOOD © 07

Areas of Obstruction in Sleep Apnea

Fig. 1. The exact location of collapse varies in different individuals and it is for that exact reason that various surgical procedures or devices fabricated to treat OSA have failed. (*Courtesy of* Mansoor Madani, DMD, MD, Bala Institute of Oral and Facial Surgery, Bala Cynwyd, PA. All rights reserved.)

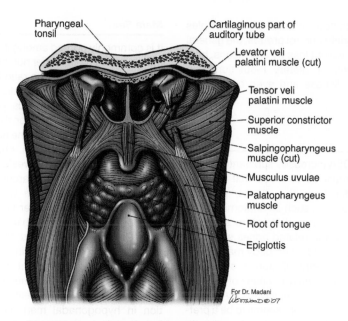

Pharyngeal tonsil

Cartilaginous part of auditory tube

Levator veli palatini muscle (cut)

Tensor veli palatini muscle

Superior constrictor muscle

Salpingopharyngeus muscle (cut)

Musculus uvulae

Palatopharyngeus muscle

Root of tongue

Epiglottis

For Dr. Madani

Musculature of the Posterior Pharynx

Fig. 2. Retropositioning of the tongue is one of the most common feature of patients with OSA, but the dimension of pharyngeal lumen and the elongation of the uvula and soft palatal draping also seem to play important roles. (*Courtesy of* Mansoor Madani, DMD, MD, Bala Institute of Oral and Facial Surgery, Bala Cynwyd, PA. All rights reserved.)

reduced by combined procedures performed on the soft palate, such as laser-assisted uvulopalatopharyngoplasty (LA-UPPP), and nasal turbinate and septal procedures, such as radioablation and septoplasty.[2,5–7]

Adding to the complexity of anatomic abnormalities causing airway obstruction, there are other factors, such as physiologic and functional impairment of the upper airway dilating muscles. Reduction of tonic and phasic contractions of these muscles during sleep has been well demonstrated. Additionally, various defective respiratory control mechanisms are found in conjunction with OSA, including impaired chemical drive, defective inspiratory load responses, and abnormal upper airway protective reflexes. These defects lead to a reduced ventilator response to hypercapnia and an elevated partial pressure of carbon dioxide in arterial blood ($PaCO_2$). However, the cause of lower chemosensitivity to carbon dioxide in patients with sleep apnea is uncertain.

Obesity

Based on the latest statistics of the World Health Organization (WHO), there are more than 1.6 billion overweight adults and at least 400 million obese individuals on earth. The WHO projects that by 2015, approximately 2.3 billion adults will be overweight and more than 700 million will be obese.

Over 20 million children younger than 5 years were overweight in 2005. The obesity rates have increased 3-fold or more since 1980 in some areas of North America, the United Kingdom, Eastern Europe, the Middle East, the Pacific Islands, Australasia, and China. There is no question that obesity and sleep apnea go hand-in-hand. Although all patients who suffer from OSA are not obese, it can easily be assumed based on many epidemiologic studies that as many as 90% of obese patients suffer from sleep apnea.[3,19–25] The exact mechanism of this relationship could be explained in numerous ways. In general, obese individual have physical changes related to their upper airway anatomy. Increased parapharyngeal fat deposition results in a smaller upper airway. This alteration in the anatomy and in the physiologic collapsibility of the upper airway are amongst several factors that influences the increased chance of OSA. Alterations in neural compensatory mechanisms that maintain airway patency and altered relationship between respiratory drive and load compensation reduce functional residual capacity of the lungs and, therefore, increased whole-body oxygen demand. Specific anatomic locations of excess fat deposition may also be important. It is possible that different types of distributions defined as cervical and truncal obesity may be more important risk factors in predictability of apnea. Although limited by small study samples and lack of appropriate control groups, the general observation is that weight loss by any means, be it surgical intervention or dietary restriction, can lessen severity of disease and even be curative in some patients.

Aging

The frequency of OSA increases substantially with age. However, it must be stressed that younger patients also suffer from this illness, possibly because of other factors, such as anatomic upper airway obstruction. Published literature supports the concept that the age-related apnea seems to plateau after 65 years and when body mass index is controlled; the severity of apnea seems to decrease with age, potentially because of survivor effects.[26,27] Anatomic susceptibility to OSA seems to worsen with aging, and there seems to be a preferential deposition of fat around the pharynx with aging, independent of systemic fat, lengthening of the soft palate, and changes in body structures surrounding the pharynx. Similar to many upper airway reflexes, the genioglossus negative pressure reflex seems to deteriorate with aging. Indeed, these anatomic and physiologic factors probably contribute to increased upper airway collapsibility with aging. Other pathophysiological factors, such as arousal threshold, appear to be less important in mediating the aging predisposition to OSA. Finally, although lung compliance is known to increase with aging, the authors are not aware of systematic studies that have assessed how loss of lung elastic recoil with aging affects upper airway mechanics.

Pregnancy and Menopause

Pregnancy has been reported to be associated with a higher prevalence of snoring, choking, and awakenings, particularly in the third trimester. Although some of the physiologic changes that accompany pregnancy (eg, higher progesterone levels and decrease in sleep time in the supine position) may protect against OSA, gestational weight gain, decrease in pharyngeal luminal size due to diffuse pharyngeal edema, effect of sleep deprivation on pharyngeal dilator muscle activity, and altered pulmonary physiology increase the tendency for disordered breathing during sleep. There is evidence that the effect of pregnancy on snoring resolves within several months after delivery. The effects of menopause and hormone therapy on OSA are also well reported in the literature.[28–37]

Male Sex

It is commonly agreed amongst most practitioners that there is a much larger number of men affected by OSA than women. The ratio between men and women in clinical-based studies ranges from 2:1 to 9:1 according to various papers. There are several possible reasons for this disparity in sex difference ratio. The first is the neck circumference and fatty deposits in the pharyngeal airways. Imaging studies have revealed that men have increased fat deposition around the pharyngeal airway as compared with women.[38–42] Tongue size also seem to be larger in men than women, contributing more readily to upper airway obstruction. One further factor is that the pharyngeal airway seems to be longer in men than in women, which may play an important role in contributing to airway collapsibility. Hormonal differences may also play a role. In fact, testosterone administration in hypogonadal men has been shown to induce sleep-disordered breathing in some patients. Truncal obesity seems to be more common in men than women and presents a much greater risk of upper airway collapsibility by reducing caudal traction and lung volume gas-exchange potential. Another factor noted in the author's center is that men seem to have more tendencies to suffer from very loud snoring, gasping for air, snorting, and having witnessed apneas, whereas women have a greater tendency to report symptoms of fatigue, nightmares, and lack of energy. It is thought that differential response of the bed partner to the symptoms of obstructive breathing during sleep may contribute to clinical under-recognition of the disorder in women. Female bed partners of male patients seem to have a lower threshold for symptom perception and reporting than male bed partners of female patients.

Familial and Genetic Predisposition

Familial susceptibility to OSA was first recognized in the 1970s by Strohl and colleagues[43] in a family with several affected individuals.[44] Since then, several large-scale studies have confirmed a role for inheritance and familial factors in the genesis of OSA. Familial susceptibility for snoring and apnea seems to increase directly with the number of affected relatives.[45]

Craniomaxillofacial morphology is a well known example of how genetic factors can influence form, shape, and size of the skeletal and soft tissue structures in the upper airway, hence, an important factor in upper airway collapsibility during sleep. Genetic predisposition to OSA could be divided into 2 types of abnormality. The first is the skeletal abnormality, including retrognathic maxilla or mandible, chin size and position, nasal shape, and so forth. The second type, inherited in some part, is the abnormalities involving the soft tissue structures, such as the soft palate and total soft-tissue–mass structures in the upper airways, and the size of the uvula and tongue and volume of the lateral parapharyngeal walls. As discussed earlier, the genetic determinants of obesity and regional fat distribution are also relevant, implicating these factors in the pathogenesis of the sleep disorder.

It is estimated that approximately one-fourth of the prevalence of OSA or an elevated apnea-hypopnea index has a genetic basis. An observation in the author's center is that over 62% of patients who complain of snoring report that one or more of their parents and siblings also snore. Examinations of the oropharyngeal, nasopharyngeal, and skeletal structures confirm the similarity of the anatomic shapes causing the snoring or OSA. However, the genetic influence is multifactorial rather than due to a single mutation or protein action. Such clustering does not warrant testing of the asymptomatic family members of a patient with snoring and OSA.

Nasal Congestion

A biologic basis for nasal congestion during sleep as a cause of obstructive apnea lies in the importance of nasal breathing to the pressure differential between the atmosphere and intrathoracic space, with increased pressure difference predisposing one to airway collapse. The importance of the role of nasal congestion in OSA is indicated by the increased frequency of snoring and sleep apnea as related to seasonal rhinitis when symptomatic, as opposed to symptom-free. Understanding the role of allergy-related nasal congestion is of particular importance, because this condition can be diminished by desensitization, allergen avoidance, or pharmacologic therapy.[46–52] Nasal congestion confers an approximately 2-fold increase in the prevalence of OSA compared with controls, regardless of the cause of nasal congestion.

Presence of postnasal drip increases surface tension of the liquid lining of the upper airway, which could influence pharyngeal patency. Patients with obstructed nasal airflow seem to be more affected because the breathing route will change to oral breathing alone, influencing the upper respiratory surface tension. Although these studies highlight a role for surface tension in OSA pathogenesis, the clinical relevance of surface tension in OSA remains less certain.[53–56]

Alcohol and Smoking

Alcohol intake can compromise breathing during sleep by acutely increasing nasal and pharyngeal resistance. The mechanism by which alcohol induces or worsens pharyngeal collapse is possibly the reduced respiratory motor output to the upper airway, resulting in hypotonia of the oropharyngeal muscles. Ingestion of alcohol before sleep has been shown to increase upper airway collapsibility and to precipitate obstructive apnea and hypopnea during sleep. It can also prolong apnea duration and worsen the severity of associated hypoxemia.[57–67]

Smoking is also considered as a risk factor for snoring and OSA. There may be several mechanisms by which smoking affects OSA, including smoking-related increases in sleep instability and airway inflammation. Sleep instability, which has been linked to OSA, may be increased by overnight reductions in nicotine blood levels. Further, a "rebound effect" may occur in which the acute effects of nicotine that favor increased upper airway tone are reversed during overnight nicotine withdrawal. In addition, smoking-related airway inflammation and disease may increase vulnerability to OSA. Smokers are believed to have 3 times more likelihood of having OSA than people who have never smoked.

SUMMARY

There is no disagreement regarding the need for early and better recognition and treatment of sleep apnea and the role that dental professionals play to facilitate diagnosis, improve patient education, and device methods to potentially address many areas of upper airway obstruction. However, critical questions remain regarding what clinical and public health approaches are needed or available to address this widespread illness in society. Dental professionals should be more vigilant in patient screening and should educate and guide their patients to seek treatment or advise them to take action, such as reducing weight and stopping smoking. Simple questions about snoring frequency and loudness, witnessed nocturnal apneas, and daytime sleepiness should become a routine component of the review of systems in the general medical history interview in dental practices.

REFERENCES

1. Madani M. Snoring and sleep apnea: a review article. Arch Iran Med 2007;10(2):215–26.
2. Madani M. Complications of laser–assisted uvulopalatopharyngoplasty (LA-UPPP) and radiofrequency

treatment of snoring and chronic nasal congestion: a 10-year review of 5,600 patients. J Oral Maxillofac Surg 2004;62:1351–62.

3. Sakakibara H, Tong M, Matsushita K, et al. Cephalometric abnormalities in non-obese and obese patients with obstructive sleep apnoea. Eur Respir J 1999;13:403–10.

4. Ephros HD, Madani M, Geller BM, et al. Developing a protocol for the surgical management of snoring and obstructive sleep apnea. Atlas Oral Maxillofac Surg Clin North Am 2007;15(2):89–100.

5. Madani M. Laser Assisted Uvulopalatopharyngoplasty (LA-UPPP) for the treatment of snoring and mild to moderate obstructive sleep apnea. Atlas Oral Maxillofac Surg Clin North Am 2007;15(2): 129–37.

6. Madani M. Radiofrequency treatment of the soft palate, nasal turbinates and tonsils for the treatment of snoring and mild to moderate obstructive sleep apnea. Atlas Oral Maxillofac Surg Clin North Am 2007;15(2):139–53.

7. Madani M. Palatal implants for treatment of habitual snoring; techniques, indications and limitations. Atlas Oral Maxillofac Surg Clin North Am 2007; 15(2):155–61.

8. Lee NR, Madani M. Genioglossus muscle advancement techniques for obstructive sleep apnea. Atlas Oral Maxillofac Surg Clin North Am 2007;15(2): 179–92.

9. Madani M. Sleep apnea: dental clinical advisor. St Louis (MO): Mosby-Elsevier; 2006. p. 27–8.

10. Davies RJ, Stradling JR. The relationship between neck circumference, radiographic pharyngeal anatomy, and the obstructive sleep apnoea syndrome. Eur Respir J 1990;3:509–14.

11. Hoffstein V, Mateika S. Differences in abdominal and neck circumferences in patients with and without obstructive sleep apnoea. Eur Respir J 1992;5:377–81.

12. Lindberg E, Gislason T. Epidemiology of sleep-related obstructive breathing. Sleep Med Rev 2000;4:411–33.

13. Stradling JR, Crosby JH. Predictors and prevalence of obstructive sleep apnea and snoring in 1001 middle aged men. Thorax 1991;46:85–90.

14. Davies RJO, Stradling JR. The epidemiology of sleep apnoea. Thorax 1996;51:S65–70.

15. Redline S. Epidemiology of sleep-disordered breathing. Semin Respir Crit Care Med 1998;19: 113–22.

16. Enright PL, Newman AB, Wahl PW, et al. Prevalence and correlates of snoring and observed apneas in 5,201 older adults. Sleep 1996;19:531–8.

17. Young T, Peppard PE. Epidemiology of obstructive sleep apnea. In: McNicholas WT, Phillipson EA, editors. Breathing disorders in sleep. London: W.B. Saunders; 2002. p. 31–43.

18. Phoha RL, Dickel MJ, Mosko SS. Preliminary longitudinal assessment of sleep in the elderly. Sleep 1990; 13:425–9.

19. Shelton KE, Woodson H, Gay S, et al. Pharyngeal fat in obstructive sleep apnea. Am Rev Respir Dis 1993; 148:462–6.

20. Mokdad AH, Serdula MK, Dietz WH, et al. The spread of the obesity epidemic in the United States, 1991–1998. JAMA 1999;282:1519–22.

21. Madani M, Madani F. The pandemic of obesity and its relationship to sleep apnea. Atlas Oral Maxillofac Surg Clin North Am 2007;15(2):81–8.

22. Carlson JT, Hedner JA, Ejnell H, et al. High prevalence of hypertension in sleep apnea patients independent of obesity. Am J Respir Crit Care Med 1994;150:72–7.

23. Strobel RJ, Rosen RC. Obesity and weight loss in obstructive sleep apnea: a critical review. Sleep 1996;19:104–15.

24. Millman RP, Carlisle CC, McGarvey ST, et al. Body fat distribution and sleep apnea severity in women. Chest 1995;107:362–6.

25. Mortimore IL, Marshall I, Wraith PK, et al. Neck and total body fat deposition in nonobese and obese patients with sleep apnea compared with that in control subjects. Am J Respir Crit Care Med 1998; 157:280–3.

26. Strohl K, Redline S. Recognition of obstructive sleep apnea. Am J Respir Crit Care Med 1996;154: 274–89.

27. Bixler E, Vgontzas A, Ten Have T, et al. Effects of age on sleep apnea in men. Am J Respir Crit Care Med 1998;157:144–8.

28. Krystal A, Edinger J, Wohlgemuth W, et al. Sleep in peri-menopausal and post-menopausal women. Sleep Med Rev 1998;2:243–53.

29. Wilhoit S, Suratt P. Obstructive sleep apnea in premenopausal women. Chest 1987;91:654–8.

30. Chakravarti S, Collins WP, Forecast JD, et al. Hormone profiles after the menopause. Br Med J 1976;2:211–8.

31. Trevoux R, De Brux J, Castanier M, et al. Endometrium and plasma hormone profile in the peri-menopause and post-menopause. Maturitas 1986;8: 309–26.

32. Toth MJ, Tchernof A, Sites CK, et al. Effect of menopausal status on body composition and abdominal fat. Int J Obes Relat Metab Disord 2000;24:226–31.

33. Espeland MA, Stefanick ML, Kritz-Silverstein D, et al. Effect of postmenopausal hormone therapy on body weight and waist and hip girths. J Clin Endocrinol Metab 1997;82:1549–56.

34. Matthews KA, Kuller LH, Winng RR, et al. Prior to use of estrogen replacement therapy, are users healthier than nonusers? Am J Epidemiol 1996;143:971–8.

35. Manson JE, Martin KA. Postmenopausal hormone-replacement therapy. N Engl J Med 2001;345:34–40.

36. Young T. Menopause, hormone replacement therapy, and sleep-disordered breathing: are we ready for the heat? Am J Respir Crit Care Med 2001;163:597–601.

37. Shaver JL, Zenk SN. Sleep disturbance in menopause. J Womens Health Gend Based Med 2000;9:109–18.

38. Popovic RM, White DP. Upper airway muscle activity in normal women: influence of hormonal status. J Appl Physiol 1998;84:1055–62.

39. Schwab RJ. Sex differences and sleep apnoea. Thorax 1999;54:284–5.

40. Ware JC, McBrayer RH, Scott JA. Influence of sex and age on duration and frequency of sleep apnea events. Sleep 2000;23:165–70.

41. Leech J, Onal E, Dulberg C, et al. A comparison of men and women with occlusive sleep apnea syndrome. Chest 1988;94:983–8.

42. Whittle AT, Marshall I, Mortimore IL, et al. Neck soft tissue and fat distribution: comparison between normal men and women by magnetic resonance imaging. Thorax 1999;54:323–8.

43. Strohl KP, Saunders NA, Feldman NT, et al. Obstructive sleep apnea in family members. N Engl J Med 1978;299:969–73.

44. Baumel M, Maislin G, Pack A. Population and occupational screening for obstructive sleep apnea: are we there yet? Am J Respir Crit Care Med 1997;155:9–14.

45. Redline S, Larkin E, Schluchter M, et al. Incidence of sleep disordered breathing (SDB) in a population-based sample. Sleep 2001;24:511.

46. Lindberg E, Elmsry A, Gislason T, et al. Evolution of sleep apnea syndrome in sleepy snorers: a population-based prospective study. Am J Respir Crit Care Med 1999;159:2024–7.

47. Bixler E, Vgontzas A, Lin H, et al. Prevalence of sleep-disordered breathing in women. Am J Respir Crit Care Med 2001;163:608–13.

48. Durán J, Esnaola S, Rubio R, et al. Obstructive sleep apnea–hypopnea and related clinical features in a population-based sample of subjects aged 30 to 70 yr. Am J Respir Crit Care Med 2001;163:685–9.

49. Redline S, Tosteson T, Tishler PV, et al. Studies in the genetics of obstructive sleep apnea: familial aggregation of symptoms associated with sleep-related breathing disturbances. Am Rev Respir Dis 1992;145:440–4.

50. Blakley BW, Mahowald MW. Nasal resistance and sleep apnea. Laryngoscope 1987;97:752–4.

51. Metes A, Ohki M, Cole P, et al. Snoring, apnea and nasal resistance in men and women. J Otolaryngol 1991;20:57–61.

52. Miljeteig H, Hoffstein V, Cole P. The effect of unilateral and bilateral nasal obstruction on snoring and sleep apnea. Laryngoscope 1992;102:1150–2.

53. Young TB, Finn L, Kim HC. Nasal obstruction as a risk factor for sleep-disordered breathing. J Allergy Clin Immunol 1997;99:S757–62.

54. McNicholas WT, Tarlo S, Cole P, et al. Obstructive apneas during sleep in patients with seasonal allergic rhinitis. Am Rev Respir Dis 1982;126:625–8.

55. Zwillich CW, Pickett C, Hanson FN, et al. Disturbed sleep and prolonged apnea during nasal obstruction in normal men. Am Rev Respir Dis 1981;124:158–60.

56. Shepard JW Jr, Burger CD. Nasal and oral flow–volume loops in normal subjects and patients with obstructive sleep apnea. Am Rev Respir Dis 1990;142:1288–93.

57. Young T, Finn L, Palta M. Chronic nasal congestion at night is a risk factor for snoring in a population-based cohort study. Arch Intern Med 2001;161:1514–9.

58. Kirkness JP, Madronio M, Stavrinou R, et al. Relationship between surface tension of upper airway lining liquid and upper airway collapsibility during sleep in obstructive sleep apnea hypopnea syndrome. J Appl Physiol 2003;95:1761–6.

59. Jokic R, Klimaszewski A, Mink J, et al. Surface tension forces in sleep apnea: the role of a soft tissue lubricant: a randomized double-blind, placebo-controlled trial. Am J Respir Crit Care Med 1998;157:1522–5.

60. Kirkness JP, Madronio M, Stavrinou R, et al. Surface tension of upper airway mucosal lining liquid in obstructive sleep apnea/hypopnea syndrome. Sleep 2005;28:457–63.

61. Verma M, Seto-Poon M, Wheatley JR, et al. Influence of breathing route on upper airway lining liquid surface tension in humans. J Physiol 2006;574:859–66.

62. Scanlan MF, Roebuck T, Little PJ, et al. Effect of moderate alcohol upon obstructive sleep apnoea. Eur Respir J 2000;16:909–13.

63. Taasan VC, Block AJ, Boysen PG, et al. Alcohol increases sleep apnea and oxygen desaturation in asymptomatic men. Am J Med 1981;71:240–5.

64. Tsutsumi W, Miyazaki S, Itasaka Y, et al. Influence of alcohol on respiratory disturbance during sleep. Psychiatry Clin Neurosci 2000;54:332–3.

65. Berry RB, Desa MM, Light RW. Effect of ethanol on the efficacy of nasal continuous positive airway pressure as a treatment for obstructive sleep apnea. Chest 1991;99:339–43.

66. Scrima L, Hartman PG, Hiller FC. Effect of three alcohol doses on breathing during sleep in 30–49 year old nonobese snorers and nonsnorers. Alcohol Clin Exp Res 1989;13:420–7.

67. Wetter DW, Young TB, Bidwell TR, et al. Smoking as a risk factor for sleep-disordered breathing. Arch Intern Med 1994;154:2219–24.

Evaluation of the Obstructive Sleep Apnea Patient and Management of Snoring

N. Ray Lee, DDS[a,b,*]

KEYWORDS

- Obstructive sleep apnea • Management of snoring
- Daytime sleepiness • Apnea-hypopnea index

Since the first published reports of excessive daytime sleepiness and failed respiratory events during sleep,[1–3] there has been an impressive quest for knowledge and an exponential growth in public demand for answers in the treatment of sleep apnea. In 1990, there were 110,000 office visits for sleep apnea complaints, and by 1998, 1.3 million annual office visits were recorded.[4] Today, thanks to many clinical and academic researchers, specialty societies, such as the American Academy of Sleep Medicine (AASM) and the American Academy of Dental Sleep Medicine, and the multitudes of patients willing to be study participants, progress continues in evaluating and managing obstructive sleep apnea (OSA). Recently, the AASM, published a comprehensive clinical guideline for the evaluation, management, and long-term care of OSA in adults.[5] The guideline was designed to assist sleep-medicine specialists, surgeons, dentists, and primary care providers who care for patients with OSA, by providing a comprehensive strategy for the evaluation, management, and long-term care of adults with OSA. The major objective of this article is to provide a practical strategy for the systematic evaluation of the OSA patient. The article also discusses the management of snoring. The presented strategy is based upon review of the current literature, the principles set forth in the AASM clinical guideline publication, and the author's personal experience.

INITIAL EVALUATION

It is essential that the presence and severity of OSA be determined before initiating any therapy. This important diagnostic strategy (1) facilitates identification of those patients at risk of developing complications of sleep apnea, (2) guides selection of appropriate treatment, and (3) provides a baseline to measure the effectiveness of subsequent treatment.[5] When the patient presents for a surgical consultation, a comprehensive evaluation should be completed. Major components of the evaluation include a comprehensive history, physical examination, indicated imaging studies, and evaluation of the results of sleep studies.

Health History

A thorough sleep-specific history and comprehensive medical history are essential components of the evaluation. A systematic approach to data acquisition for OSA assessment is crucial before referral to a sleep center for evaluation polysomnography (PSG). The primary indication for initiation of the evaluation process is the presence

a Department of Oral and Maxillofacial Surgery, Medical College of Virginia, Virginia Commonwealth University, 520 North 12th Street, Richmond, VA 23298, USA
b Private Practice, Oyster Point Oral and Facial Surgery, 11842 Rock Landing Drive, Suite 105, Newport News, VA 23606, USA
*Corresponding author.
E-mail address: reyzor1@aol.com

Oral Maxillofacial Surg Clin N Am 21 (2009) 377–387
doi:10.1016/j.coms.2009.09.002

of OSA symptoms. Symptom discovery should begin with a detailed patient health history that includes questions about such specific OSA symptoms as loud snoring (presence and character), witnessed apneas, gasping/choking during sleep, excessive daytime sleepiness, and perceived quality and quantity of sleep (**Fig. 1**). It is therefore of utmost importance to include the patient's bed partner in symptom discovery.

Questionnaires that assess the presence of OSA signs should be included in the medical record, as they are essential to the development of a subjective analysis of the patient's complaints and form a basis for determining associated quality-of-life issues. These questionnaires should be completed during the initial evaluation, and repeated after 4 to 6 months of treatment to document subjective improvement in patient complaints.

Valid and reliable measurement tools are available to evaluate sleepiness and quality of life in OSA patients. The Epworth Sleepiness Scale, developed by Murray Johns at the Epworth Sleep Center, Richmond, Victoria, Australia,[6,7] is an excellent measure of the patient's general level of daytime sleepiness. The scale is easy to use. Patients simply score their likelihood of falling asleep in eight different situations (**Fig. 2**). The Calgary Sleep Apnea Quality of Life Index[8,9] and the Functional Outcomes of Sleep Questionnaire[10] are two sleep-specific quality-of-life questionnaires that may also be used. Although quantitative postoperative analysis using a reduction in the apnea-hypopnea index (AHI) has been the standard measure to judge successful surgical outcomes, the value of the subjective assessment of postoperative sleepiness and quality of life, derived from these surveys, should not be underestimated. Thus, each of the listed measurement tools may be useful for assessment of subjective improvement in daytime sleepiness and quality of life 4 to 6 months after surgery.

A comprehensive medical history must be obtained because OSA is associated with a wide spectrum of medical conditions. The health history reveals findings associated with obesity, hypertension, stroke, or other cardiopulmonary or neurologic conditions linked to a higher risk of OSA. The health history also identifies characteristics of comorbidities associated with OSA that are

CHIEF COMPLAINT: _____

SLEEP HISTORY:

Excessive daytime sleepiness? :   __No   __Yes: __Mild   __Moderate   __Severe
Witnessed apneic episodes? :   __No   __Yes
Gasping/choking at night? :   __No   __Yes
Loud snoring: __No   __Yes: __Mild   __Moderate   __Severe
Non-refreshing sleep? :   __No   __Yes

POLYSOMNOGRAPHY: Date _____ AHI: _____ Low SaO2: _____

CPAP THERAPY:

Attempted to use CPAP: __No   __Yes   CPAP Pressure: _____
Able to tolerate/adhere to CPAP therapy?:   __No   __Yes
Unable to adhere to CPAP therapy because:
__Initial intolerance __Mask fit problems__Pressure intolerance __Skin irritations __Nasal symptoms
__Claustrophobia __Unintentional mask removal __Machine noise __Other:_____

ORAL APPLIANCE THERAPY: __No __Yes Dates of Use:_____

PAST SURGICAL HISTORY (Including dates of surgery):

Tonsillectomy/Adenoidectomy: _____ Nasal Surgery:_____ Uvulopalatoplasty: _____
Other Procedures:_____
Post-Treatment Polysomnography: Date _____ AHI: _____ Low SaO2: _____
Any treatment-related symptoms or complications?: _____

PAST MEDICAL HISTORY:

Hypertension: __No __Yes   Diabetes: __No __Yes Irregular Heart Beat: __No __Yes
Heart Failure: __No __Yes   Heart Attack:__No __Yes Stroke: __No __Yes

Any significant conditions including cardiovascular, endocrine, pulmonary, neurologic, hepatic, renal or psychiatric disease?

_____

CURRENT MEDICATIONS AND DOSES:

_____

Fig. 1. Form for documenting health history at OSA consultation visit.

Name: _____ Today's date: _____

Your age (Yrs): _____ Your sex (Male = M, Female = F): _____

How likely are you to doze off or fall asleep in the following situations, in contrast to feeling just tired?

This refers to your usual way of life in recent times.

Even if you haven't done some of these things recently try to work out how they would have affected you.

Use the following scale to choose the **most appropriate number** for each situation:

0 = would **never** doze
1 = **slight chance** of dozing
2 = **moderate chance** of dozing
3 = **high chance** of dozing

It is important that you answer each question as best you can.

Situation   **Chance of Dozing (0-3)**

Sitting and reading   _____   ___

Watching TV   _____   ___

Sitting, inactive in a public place (e.g. a theatre or a meeting)   _____   ___

As a passenger in a car for an hour without a break   _____   ___

Lying down to rest in the afternoon when circumstances permit _____   ___

Sitting and talking to someone   _____   ___

Sitting quietly after a lunch without alcohol   _____   ___

In a car, while stopped for a few minutes in the traffic _____

THANK YOU FOR YOUR COOPERATION

© **M.W. Johns 1990-97**

Fig. 2. Questionnaire for Epworth Sleepiness Scale. (*Courtesy of* M.W. Johns MD, Melbourne, Australia; with permission. © Copyright M.W. Johns, 1990–1997.)

essential to further medical referrals and the formulation of a treatment plan. If surgical treatment of OSA is indicated, the status of any significant medical conditions must be defined (1) to determine if the patient is a candidate for surgery, (2) to determine what can be done to improve the patient's condition before surgery, and (3) to develop a plan for intraoperative and postoperative management of each significant medical condition.

The patient should also be questioned about previous treatment of OSA and past response to therapy. This should include both the patient's subjective and objective (eg, posttreatment PSG) response to therapy. Patients should also be questioned about any treatment-related adverse outcomes or complications of previous therapy. To complete a comprehensive evaluation of the patient's history, previous surgical treatments and sleep study reports should ideally be requested and reviewed before the initial office visit. Additionally, documentation of the medical reason for continuous positive airway pressure (CPAP) failure (preferably from the sleep physician), should be obtained, as it may be required for preauthorization of future surgical procedures.

When the initial consultation appointment is scheduled, the patient should be instructed to send (or bring with them to the consultation visit) the reports of all previous sleep studies. These reports are essential to establish the presence and severity of OSA. It is likely that the patient has had a CPAP titration performed and the titration results will give an indication of the effectiveness of CPAP if the patient is compliant with CPAP therapy. Furthermore, if the patient has undergone treatment of OSA, posttreatment sleep studies may have been completed to assess the result of therapy. The most recent sleep study should accurately reflect the patient's current status. If significant time has elapsed since the last study or if the patient's symptoms (eg, daytime sleepiness) have significantly changed (especially worsened), a repeat sleep study is indicated to accurately assess the current severity of OSA.

Physical Examination

For each patient, the clinician should perform a comprehensive head and neck examination and assess the respiratory, cardiovascular, and neurologic systems.[5] The process of identifying characteristics consistent with OSA from the physical examination is well described in the literature.[11] **Fig. 3** outlines a sample OSA patient form, which may be used as a guide for capturing the essential elements of the OSA physical examination during the consultation visit. Such physical findings as obesity (body mass index [BMI] ≥ 30 kg/m^2), craniofacial abnormality (eg, mandibular retrognathia), increased neck circumference (>17 in in men; >16 in in women), anatomic nasal airway deformity (eg, turbinate hypertrophy, nasoseptal deviation, polyps), elongated/enlarged soft palate, high-arched/narrow palate, hypertrophic tonsils and adenoids, lateral peritonsillar narrowing, and macroglossia are all suggestive of OSA.[5]

Special attention should be paid to potential sites of upper airway obstruction during the examination. The nasal complex can be evaluated by external inspection and intranasal examination by speculum or nasopharyngoscopy. The tonsils, tonsillar pillars, tongue, uvula, soft palate and hard palate can be assessed by direct examination and the anatomic findings can be graded, using the Friedman Staging System (FSS).[12–14] The FSS (**Table 1**) consists of three components of evaluation including (1) Friedman palate position (FPP) (**Fig. 4**), (2) tonsil size (**Fig. 5**), and (3) BMI. The FPP is a modification of the assessment proposed by Mallampati,[15] which is used to evaluate the relationship between the tongue and oral cavity, as an indicator of the difficulty of endotracheal intubation. In the Mallampati evaluation, the patient protrudes the tongue, in contrast to the FPP, where the tongue is evaluated in a natural,

relaxed position similar to the position achieved during sleep. The anatomic findings of the FSS are used to predict the severity of sleep-disordered breathing.[12] The FSS has also been shown to be a good predictor of the effectiveness of uvulopalatopharyngoplasty for the treatment of OSA.[16] In fact, the anatomy-based FSS predicted uvulopalatopharyngoplasty outcome better then the AHI severity-based staging system. Individuals classified as stage I are effectively treated by uvulopalatopharyngoplasty, in contrast to stage II and III patients, who are best treated by surgical procedures, such as maxillomandibular advancement, that treat tongue base obstruction.[14]

In addition to direct visual examination, endoscopic examination (fiber optic nasopharyngoscopy) of the upper airway may be of benefit to aid in seeing the upper airway and identifying the site or sites of pharyngeal collapse and obstruction.

Imaging Studies

Imaging studies, including a panoramic radiograph and lateral cephalometric radiograph, should also be part of the initial evaluation. Radiographs are inexpensive and readily available, making them a valuable component of the diagnostic evaluation. The cephalometric radiograph is a static two-dimensional interpretation of the three-dimensional upper airway, with standards for uniform interpretation. Exposure is always at end expiration, and each exposure has a standard position and distance from the central beam to the target.

A cephalometric radiograph offers the unique quantification of craniofacial anatomy necessary in the treatment of craniofacial deformities and OSA. DeBerry-Borowiecki and colleagues[17] concluded that cephalometric analysis is useful in conjunction with head and neck examination, PSG studies, and endoscopic studies to evaluate patients with OSA, and in planning surgical treatment for improvement of upper airway patency. Jamieson and coworkers[18] demonstrated the following characteristics on cephalometric examination in patients with OSA: a normally positioned maxilla, retroposition of the mandible, and abnormal cranial base flexure, with a smaller than expected (ie, more acute) nasion-sella-basion angle. The combined effect of a normally positioned maxilla and retroposition of the mandible reduces the space occupied by soft tissue anchored on the skull and mandible.

While a cephalogram should be included in the diagnostic armamentarium for upper airway anatomy evaluation in patients with OSA, its

Vital signs: Blood Pressure: _____   Pulse: _____

General: Weight (lbs): _____   Height (inches): _____   BMI: _____   Neck Circumference (inches): _____

Face: Frontal view (Lower Facial Height): ___ Normal   ___ Increased   ___ Decreased
Profile view: ___ Straight/Orthognathic   ___ Convex/Retrognathic   ___ Concave/Prognathic

Neck: Tenderness, masses or cervical lymphadenopathy?: ___ No   ___ Yes Trachea midline?: ___ No   ___ Yes
Tenderness or enlargement of salivary glands?: ___ No   ___ Yes
Hypertrophy or enlargement of Thyroid?: ___ No   ___ Yes

Nasal Complex:

	None	Mild	Moderate	Severe
Subjective obstruction:	___	___	___	___
Inferior turbinate hypertrophy:	___	___	___	___
Nasal complex to facial midline:	___	___	___	___
Septal Deviation:	___	___	___	___
Nasopharynx:	___	___	___	___

Alar base width: _____ (mm)

Oropharynx
Hard Palate: ___ Normal   ___ Abnormal   Findings: _____
Palatal Position (free margin): _____
Normal position   ___ Moderately low, but visible on phonation   ___ Extremely low, not visible on phonation
Uvula: ___ Normal   ___ Healed UPPP   ___ Mod. Enlarged   ___ Markedly Enlarged
Pillar Mucosa: ___ Normal (< 5mm)   ___ Mildly Wide   ___ Mod. Wide (5-10mm)   ___ Markedly Wide (>10mm)
Tonsil Size: ___ Removed   ___ Size 1   ___ Size 2   ___ Size 3   ___ Size 4

Oropharyngeal Space:
Width: ___ Normal   ___ Mildly Compromised   ___ Moderately Compromised   ___ Markedly Compromised
Depth: ___ Normal   ___ Mildly Compromised   ___ Moderately Compromised   ___ Markedly Compromised
Posterior Pharyngeal Wall: ___ Normal   ___ Mildly wrinkled   ___ Moderately wrinkled   ___ Markedly wrinkled
Oropharynx lateral wall bulge: ___ None   ___ Mild   ___ Moderate   ___ Marked

Friedman Palate Position: ___ Grade I   ___ Grade II   ___ Grade III   ___ Grade IV
(modified Malampati)
Friedman Staging System: ___ Stage I   ___ Stage II   ___ Stage III   ___ Stage IV

Temporomandibular Joints (inspection, auscultation and palpation):
Audible crepitus or clicking: ___ None   ___ Right TMJ   ___ Left TMJ   ___ Both
Palpable crepitus or clicking: ___ None   ___ Right TMJ   ___ Left TMJ   ___ Both
Palpation tenderness of condyles: ___ None   ___ Right TMJ   ___ Left TMJ   ___ Both
Maximum Mandibular Opening: _____ (mm)
Right lateral excursive movement: _____ (mm)   Left lateral excursive movement: _____ (mm)

Muscle Pain-Palpation Tenderness:

	None	Mild	Moderate	Severe
Right masseter muscle:	___	___	___	___
Left masseter muscle:	___	___	___	___
Right temporalis muscle:	___	___	___	___

	None	Mild	Moderate	Severe
Left temporalis muscle:	___	___	___	___
SCM muscle:	___	___	___	___
Trapezius muscle:	___	___	___	___

Cranial Nerve V: Neurosensory deficit(s)?
___ No   ___ Yes: Site(s) and Findings: _____

Cranial nerve VII: Motor weakness?
___ No   ___ Yes: Site(s) and Findings: _____

Facial/Dental Symmetry
Maxillary midline to facial midline: ___ Coincident   ___ Right: _____ (mm)   ___ Left: _____ (mm)
Mandibular midline to facial midline: ___ Coincident   ___ Right: _____ (mm)   ___ Left: _____ (mm)
Chin to facial midline: ___ Coincident   ___ Right: _____ (mm)   ___ Left: _____ (mm)
Vertical asymmetry/gonial angles/inferior borders of the mandible: ___ Coincident   right: _____ (mm)   left: _____ (mm)
Occlusal Cant present?: ___ None   ___ Yes: Canine: _____ (mm)   1st molar: _____ (mm)

Lip/Tooth Relations:
Maxillary incisor exposure with upper lip in repose: _____ (mm)
Maxillary incisor exposure when smiling: _____ (mm)
Interlabial gap: _____ (mm)
Dental Crowding: ___ None   ___ Yes: Findings: _____

Occlusion (Angle Classification):
Right maxillary canine: ___ I   ___ II   ___ III
Left maxillary canine: ___ I   ___ II   ___ III
Right mandibular first molar: ___ I   ___ II   ___ III
Left mandibular first molar: ___ I   ___ II   ___ III
Overjet: _____ (mm)   Overbite: _____ (mm)   Open bite: ___ None   ___ Yes: _____ (mm)
Attrition of dentition: ___ None   ___ Mild   ___ Moderate   ___ Severe

Teeth, Gingiva, and Lips:
Oral Hygiene: ___ Good   ___ Fair   ___ Poor
Caries: ___ None   ___ Mild   ___ Moderate   ___ Severe
Periodontitis: ___ None   ___ Mild   ___ Moderate   ___ Severe
Edentulism: ___ Full complement of teeth   ___ Partial Edentulism   ___ Complete Edentulism
Lip Mucosa: ___ Normal without lesions

Fig. 3. Form for documenting physical examination at OSA consultation visit.

Table 1
Friedman staging system

	Friedman Palate Position	Tonsil Size	Body Mass Index
Stage I	1	3, 4	<40
	2	3, 4	<40
Stage II	1, 2	1, 2	<40
	3, 4	3, 4	<40
Stage III	3	0, 1, 2	<40
	4	0, 1, 2	<40
Stage IV	1, 2, 3, 4	1, 2, 3, 4	>40

All patients with significant craniofacial or anatomic deformities.

Modified from Friedman M, Ibrahim H, Bass L. Clinical staging for sleep-disordered breathing. Otolaryngol Head Neck Surg 2002;127(1):13–21; with permission.

limitations should also be noted. Because the cephalogram is a two-dimensional study of three-dimensional anatomy, it does not provide accurate assessment of upper airway volume or of the effects of tonsillar hypertrophy or other lateral soft tissue on the function of the upper airway.

Other imaging studies, such as CT, MRI, and Doppler analysis, may also be useful, and details of these procedures will be covered in another article.

Polysomnography

Not all individuals who snore or are sleepy adults have OSA. Middle-aged adults snore 30% to 50% of the time, and more than 30% of adults report excessive daytime sleepiness.[19,20] In a retrospective analysis, Deegan and McNicholas[21] reported that among 250 consecutive patients referred to a sleep center with snoring as the

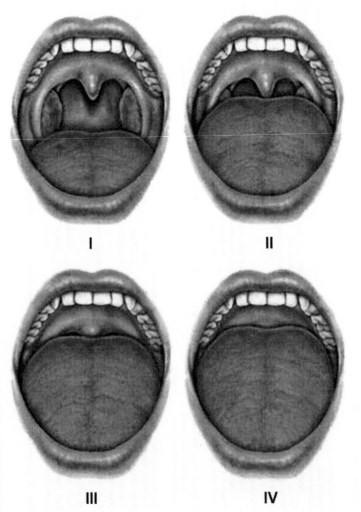

I   II

III   IV

Fig. 4. The Friedman palate position is based on visualization of structures in the mouth with the mouth open widely without protrusion of the tongue. Palate grade I allows the observer to visualize the entire uvula and tonsils. Grade II allows visualization of the uvula but not the tonsils. Grade III allows visualization of the soft palate but not the uvula. Grade IV allows visualization of the hard palate only. (*From* Friedman M, Ibrahim H, Joseph NJ. Staging of obstructive sleep apnea/hypopnea syndrome: a guide to appropriate treatment. Laryngoscope. Mar 2004;114(3):455; with permission).

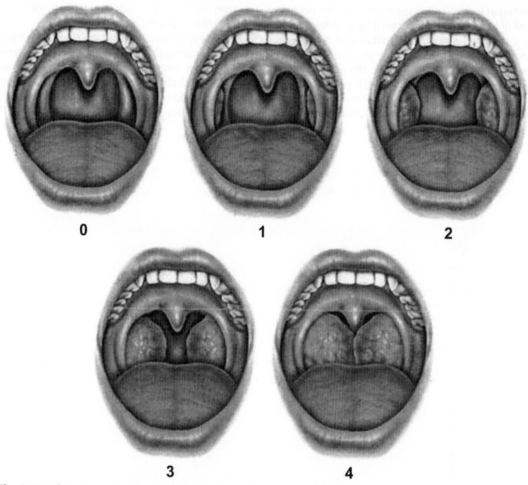

0   **1**   **2**

3   **4**

Fig. 5. Tonsil size is graded from **0** to **4**. Tonsil size **0** denotes surgically removed tonsils. Size **1** implies tonsils hidden within the pillars. Tonsil size **2** implies the tonsils extending to the pillars. Size **3** tonsils are beyond the pillars but not to the midline. Tonsil size **4** implies that tonsils extend to the midline. (*From* Friedman M, Ibrahim H, Joseph NJ. Staging of obstructive sleep apnea/hypopnea syndrome: a guide to appropriate treatment. Laryngoscope. Mar 2004;114(3):455; with permission).

predictive symptom of OSA, the calculated positive predictive value (PPV) for OSA was only 0.63 and the negative predictive value (NPV) was only 0.56. In another study, Hessel and de Vries[22] evaluated the diagnostic value of witnessed apneas and hypersomnia in 380 patients referred for a sleep study with problem snoring, and found 54% of the 380 patients had OSA (as defined by an AHI >15).

It is the conclusion of the AASM that clinical impression alone (or categorization based solely on symptoms) lacks the accuracy required for accurate diagnosis of OSA, and objective testing is also needed.[4] Since the early descriptions of PSG findings by Gastaut,[23,24] Jung and Kuhlo,[25] and others,[26,27] the in-laboratory nocturnal PSG has been the objective gold standard for modern diagnosis of OSA.

PSG evaluates sleep-disordered breathing, sleep architecture, and oxygen desaturations. A typical 8-hour nocturnal laboratory PSG involves measurement of multiple channels of physiologic parameters, including electroencephalogram, electrooculography, chin movements, leg movement via electromyography, ECG, heart rate, respiratory effort, chest wall movement, abdominal wall movement, airflow, and oxygen saturations. As these physiologic parameters are scored, a sleep technologist documents body position.[28,29] A board-certified sleep-medicine physician then interprets the test recording and scoring data to issue a report addressing the OSA diagnosis.

The primary measure of sleep-disordered breathing is the AHI, which is the number of apneas and hypopneas per hour of sleep. An apnea is defined as an interruption of airflow lasting at least 10 seconds in adults or the equivalent of two breaths in children (**Fig. 6**). A hypopnea is a specified reduction in airflow and an associated oxygen desaturation or arousal, lasting at least 10 seconds in adults or the equivalent of two breaths in children. The AHI is the primary measure used to determine the severity of OSA and effectiveness of treatment. OSA is classified as mild (AHI 5–15), moderate (AHI 15–30) and severe (AHI ≥ 30).[29]

If apnea is observed during the diagnostic PSG (AHI of 40 during the first 2 hours), CPAP therapy can then be initiated. This technique is termed a split-night study (initial diagnostic PSG followed by CPAP titration during PSG on the same night). A split-night study is acceptable only if CPAP

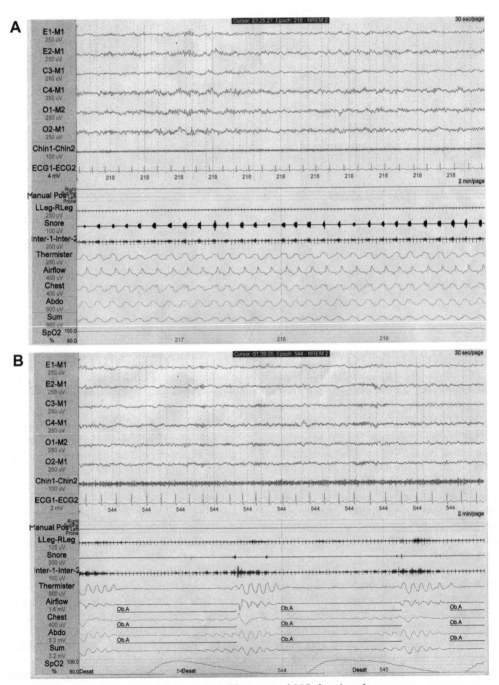

Fig. 6. (*A*) Nocturnal PSG showing simple snoring. (*B*) Nocturnal PSG showing sleep apnea.

titration lasts longer than 3 hours and results in a PSG parameter document demonstrating that CPAP nearly eliminates the respiratory events during rapid eye movement (REM) and non-REM sleep, including when the patient is in a supine position.[4]

DIAGNOSIS

The findings of the history, physical examination, PSG, and imaging studies help the surgeon judge upper airway stability within the nasopharynx, oropharynx, and hypopharynx. This judgment— along with the comorbidity findings—form the basis for a definitive treatment plan.

THE SIMPLE SNORER

If the PSG interpretation is negative for sleep-related breathing disorder—rendering a diagnosis of simple snoring—options for treatment of simple snoring should be discussed with the patient. Indications for treatment of simple snoring are clearly expressed by the patient's desire to improve his or her quality of life by eradicating this potentially socially crippling disorder. As outlined by Luqaresi,[30] simple snoring also can play a clinically significant role in systemic blood pressure fluctuations.

To achieve a successful outcome in either patients with OSA or the simple snorer, the nasal airway must be patent and without airflow limitation. This can be accomplished pharmacologically in the majority of patients. However, surgical correction may be necessary if anatomic findings compromise airflow in the nasal airway.

There are three categories of treatment options to consider when developing a comprehensive treatment for simple snoring: patient-administered interventions; nonsurgical interventions; and surgical interventions. A technical discussion of each of these categories is beyond the scope of this article. However, choices within each category are presented below.

Patient-administered Interventions

Patient-administered interventions begin with sleep-position evaluation; avoiding the supine position may diminish the snore.[31] Another effective patient-administered intervention is weight loss. Because there are strong epidemiologic links to excessive weight and increased neck circumference and sleep-related breathing disorder symptoms, part of patient-administered intervention should include emphasis on nutritional, well-balanced meal and exercise plans.

Nonsurgical Interventions

The most popular nonsurgical intervention is a dental appliance, the mandibular repositioning appliance. Effectiveness of this treatment—with few negative side effects—has been validated in the literature, with lack of patient compliance the major factor in treatment failure. Although somewhat impractical, CPAP is another effective nonsurgical intervention. While 100% effective, patients rarely accept CPAP treatment for simple snoring.

Surgical Interventions

Surgical interventions for the treatment of simple snoring include uvulopalatopharyngoplasty,[32] laser-assisted uvulopalatopharyngoplasty,[33] palatal suspension via a lateral inversion flap,[34] and other cautery-assisted palatal-stiffening procedures.[35] Successful surgical outcomes have also been demonstrated with less invasive intrapalatal procedures, such as injection snoreplasty,[36] radiofrequency thermal ablation,[37] coblation, and palatal implants.[38]

While treatment selection for the simple snorer is complex and multifactorial, the objective remains the same: to improve upper airway airflow. Ultimately, while snoring may not be cured with either a single or series of treatments, it may be controlled with intermittent maintenance therapy.

SUMMARY

Surgical reconstruction of the upper airway for the treatment of OSA continues to be an evolutionary journey, with focus on site-specific upper airway anatomic correction. The debate over maxillomandibular advancement versus multistage intrapharyngeal procedures in the surgical treatment of moderate OSA will demand continued medical evidence based on scientific research and published studies. Perhaps a universally accepted surgical algorithm for the treatment of OSA will be the outcome of such research. Regardless, oral and maxillofacial surgeons today play a vital role in successful surgical treatment of patients with OSA.

REFERENCES

1. Roxburgh F, Collis A. Notes on a case of acromegaly. Br Med J 1986;2:63–5.
2. Canton R. Case of narcolepsy. Clin Soc Trans 1889; 22:133–7.
3. Morison A. Somnolence with cyanosis cured by massage. Practitioner 1889;42:277–81.

4. Kushida CA, Littner MR, Morgenthaler T, et al. Practice parameters for the indications for polysomnography and related procedures: an update for 2005. Sleep 2005;28(4):499–521.

5. Epstein LJ, Kristo D, Strollo PJ, et al. Clinical guideline for the evaluation, management and long-term care of obstructive sleep apnea in adults. J Clin Sleep Med 2009;5(3):263–76.

6. Johns MN. New method for measuring daytime sleepiness: the Epworth Sleepiness Scale. Sleep 1991;14:540–5.

7. Johns MW. Reliability and factor analysis of the Epworth Sleepiness Scale. Sleep 1992;15(4):376–81.

8. Flemons WW, Reimer MA. Development of a disease-specific health-related quality of life questionnaire for sleep apnea. Am J Respir Crit Care Med 1998;158:494–503.

9. Flemons WW, Reimer MA. Measurement properties of the Calgary sleep apnea quality of life index. Am J Respir Crit Care Med 2002;159:159–64.

10. Weaver TE, Laizner AM, Evans LK, et al. An instrument to measure functional status outcomes for disorders of excessive sleepiness. Sleep 1997;20(10):835–43.

11. Lee NR. Surgical evaluation for reconstruction of the upper airway. Oral Maxillofacial Surg Clin North Am 2002;14:351–7.

12. Friedman M, Tanyeri H, La Rosa M, et al. Clinical predictors of obstructive sleep apnea. Laryngoscope 1999;109(12):1901–7.

13. Friedman M, Ibrahim H, Bass L. Clinical staging for sleep-disordered breathing. Otolaryngol Head Neck Surg 2002;127(1):13–21.

14. Friedman M, Ibrahim H, Joseph NJ. Staging of obstructive sleep apnea/hypopnea syndrome: a guide to appropriate treatment. Laryngoscope 2004;114(3):454–9.

15. Mallampati SR, Gatt SP, Gugino LD, et al. A clinical sign to predict difficult tracheal intubation: a prospective study. Can Anaesth Soc J 1985;32(4):429–34.

16. Li H-Y, Wang P-C, Lee L-A, et al. Prediction of uvulopalatoplasty outcome: anatomy-based staging system, versus severity-based staging system. Sleep 2006;29:1537–41.

17. DeBerry-Borowiecki B, Kukwa A, Blanks RH. Analysis for diagnosis and treatment of obstructive sleep apnea. Laryngoscope 1998;98:226–34.

18. Jamieson A, Guilleminault C, Partinen M, et al. Obstructive sleep apneic patients have craniomandibular abnormalities. Sleep 1986;9:469–77.

19. Netzer NC, Hoegel JJ, Loube D, et al. Prevalence of symptoms and risk of sleep apnea in primary care. Chest 2003;124(4):1406–14.

20. Young T, Shahar E, Nieto FJ, et al. Predictors of sleep-disordered breathing in community-dwelling adults: the Sleep Heart Health Study. Arch Intern Med 2002;162(8):893–900.

21. Deegan PC, McNicholas WT. Predictive value of clinical features for the obstructive sleep apnea syndrome. Eur Respir J. 1996;9(1):117–24.

22. Hessel NS, de Vries N. Diagnostic work-up of socially unacceptable snoring. II. Sleep endoscopy. Eur Arch Otohinolaryngol 2002;259(3):158–61.

23. Gastaut H, Tassinari CA, Duron B. Etude polygraphics des manifestations episodes (hypniques et respiratories) diurnes et nocturnes, du syndrome de Pickwick [Polygraphic study of the hyponea episode manifestations during sleep in the Pickwick Syndrome]. Rev Neurol 1965;112:568–79.

24. Gastaut H, Tassinari CA, Duron B. Polygraphic study of the episode diurnal and nocturnal (hypnic and respiratory) manifestations of the Pickwick syndrome. Brain Res 1967;1:167–86.

25. Jung R, Kuhlo W. Neurophysiological studies of abnormal night sleep and the Pickwickian syndrome. Prog Brain Res 1965;18:140–59.

26. Duron B, Tassinari CA. Syndrome de Pickwick et syndrome cardiorespiratory de obesite (a propos-dure observation). J Fr Med Chir Thor 1966;20:207–22.

27. Tassinari B, Bernardina D, Cirignotta F. Apneaic periods and the respiratory related arousal patterns during sleep in the Pickwick syndrome, a polygraphic study. Bulletin de Physio-pathologic Respiratoire 1972;8:1087–102.

28. Iber C, Ancoli-Israel S, Chesson A, et al. The AASM manual for the scoring of sleep and associated events: rules, terminology and technical specifications. Westchester (IL): American Academy of Sleep Medicine; 2007.

29. Sleep-related breathing disorders in adults: recommendations for syndrome definition and measurement techniques in clinical research. The report of an American Academy of Sleep Medicine Task Force. Sleep 1999;22(5):667–89.

30. Lugaresi E, Coccagna G, Cirignotta F, et al. Breathing during sleep in man in normal and pathological conditions. Adv Exp Med Biol 1978;99:35–45.

31. Hoffstein V. Snoring. Chest 1996;109(1):201–2.

32. Hicklin LA, Tostevin P, Dasan S. Retrospective survey of long-term results and patient satisfaction with uvulopalatopharyngoplasty for snoring. J Laryngol Otol 2000;114(9):675–81.

33. Maw J, Marsan J. Uvulopalatopharyngoplasty versus laser-assisted uvulopalatopharyngoplasty in the treatment of snoring. J Otolaryngol 1997;26(4):232–5.

34. Wolford LM, Mehra P. Modified uvulopalatopharyngoplasty: the lateral inversion flap technique. J Oral Maxillofac Surg 2001;59(10):1242–3.

35. Mair EA, Day RH. Cautery-assisted palatal stiffening operation. Otolaryngol Head Neck Surg. 2000; 122(4):547–56.

36. Brietzke SE, Mair EA. Injection snoreplasty: extended follow-up and new objective data. Otolaryngol Head Neck Surg 2003;128(5):605–15.

37. Powell NB, Riley RW, Troell RJ, et al. Radiofrequency volumetric tissue reduction of the palate in subjects with sleep-disordered breathing. Chest 1998;113(5):1163–74.

38. Ho WK, Wei WI, Chung KE. Managing disturbing snoring with palatal implant: a pilot study. Arch Otolaryngol Head Neck Surg 2004;130(6):753–8.

Imaging the Upper Airway in Patients with Sleep Disordered Breathing

Somsak Sittitavornwong, DDS, MS, Peter D. Waite, DDS, MD, MPH*

KEYWORDS

• OSA • Imaging • Surgical advancement • Lefort • Airway

Obstructive sleep apnea syndrome (OSAS) is an increasingly common disorder, but the etiology and actual site of obstruction often remain unknown.[1-17] The obstruction seldom is imaged or identified. It is estimated that 98% of adults with OSAS lack specific upper airway pathology of an obstructing nature, such as neoplastic lesions of the pharynx.[18,19] All surgical procedures, including palatoplasty and maxillo-mandibular osteotomies, must be directed toward the anatomic site of obstruction. Currently, it is very difficult to identify the site of obstruction in the awake, nonsupine patient. Therefore, better diagnostic methods must be developed to help direct treatment options and improve surgical outcomes. This article will help surgeons identify possible sites of obstruction and direct surgical intervention.

Upper airway imaging modalities primarily include nasopharyngoscopy, cephalometrics, computed tomography (CT), and magnetic resonance imaging (MRI). These imaging modalities have been used to study the effect of respiration, weight loss, dental appliances, and surgery on the upper airway. MRI and CT allow quantification of the airway and surrounding soft tissue structures in three dimensions.[20-38] Upper airway imaging is a valuable technique used to study the mechanisms underlying the pathogenesis, biomechanics, and efficacy of treatment options in patients with OSAS. Imaging studies provide significant insight into the static and dynamic structure, function of the upper airway, and soft-tissue structure during wakefulness and sleep.[29-31,35,36] Unfortunately, it remains difficult to understand and predict the pathophysiology of the airway in the awake patient.

High-quality imaging can be used as a clinical predictor in OSAS,[39] and there are many studies[25,40-51] that have attempted to accurately quantify the dimensions, configurations, sites of obstruction, and collapsibility of upper airways. In recent years, sleeping fiber optic endoscopy has been applied as an effective method to locate the obstruction site. This also can be a disturbance to normal sleep, however, and sometimes is refused by examinees. Most sleep centers do not perform nocturnal endoscopy routinely. Because most patients prefer radiological examinations, high-speed CT is an ideal way to locate the obstructive site.[24,25,52-56]

Novel imaging techniques using computer fluid dynamics (CFD) for evaluating the upper airway in OSAS, and possibly predicting treatment interventions are now available. This is a very complex bioengineering process using the most powerful computers, but it is a technique available in almost every major industry. This article discusses the current imaging methods as the standard of care, and introduces the application of CFD as a possible diagnostic and prognostic tool.

UAB Oral and Maxillofacial Surgery, University of Alabama Birmingham, 1530 Third Avenue South, SDB 419, Birmingham, AL 35294-0007, USA
* Corresponding author. UAB Oral and Maxillofacial Surgery, University of Alabama Birmingham, 1530 Third Avenue South, SDB 419, Birmingham, AL 35294-0007, USA
E-mail address: pwaite@uab.edu (P.D. Waite).

Oral Maxillofacial Surg Clin N Am 21 (2009) 389–402
doi:10.1016/j.coms.2009.08.004
1042-3699/09/$ – see front matter. Published by Elsevier Inc.

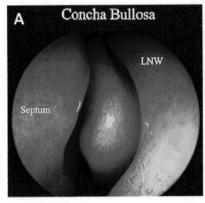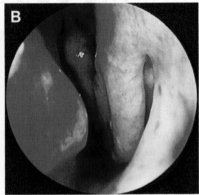

Fig. 1. (*A*) Concha bullosa. (*B*) Septal spur and deviation.

NASOPHARYNGOSCOPY

The nasal pharynx, oral pharynx, and hypopharynx can be evaluated best by endoscopic pharyngoscopy (**Fig. 1**). The goals of upper airway examination are directed at identifying traditional sites and causes of obstruction: tonsils, ectopic thyroids, radiation fibrosis, vocal cord paralysis, and lymphoma.[57] One also should try to predict the site of obstruction during sleep, such as retrognathia, which allows the tongue to fall backward during supine sleep and obstruct the airway. Another important goal is to identify areas where surgery might reduce resistance, increase size, or decrease collapsibility of the airway. Rational surgical treatment should be directed at eliminating the obstruction without creating functional impairment.

A positive Mueller's maneuver (**Table 1, Fig. 2**) is lateral collapse of the airway when the patient attempts to inhale with the nose obstructed.[58] Endoscopy easily can evaluate the shape of the airway at various locations. Retroposition of the mandible and tongue will produce a transverse airway that is diminished in the anterior–posterior dimension.[59] Nasal obstruction by itself is seldom the cause of OSAS, but it can increase negative pharyngeal pressure, leading to obstruction and collapse.[60] Catalfumo and colleaugues[61] described an epiglottic collapse that they found during Mueller maneuver in 11.5% of uvulopalatopharyngoplasty (UPPP) failures. Fiberoptic nasopharyngoscopy with Muller Maneuver (FNMM) was applied in preoperative evaluation of patients with OSAS to identify those in whom greatest pharyngeal collapse was in the region of the tonsillar fossae and soft palate. Sher and colleagues[62] reported pharyngeal changes on FNMM in patients who were considered most likely to respond to surgery and therefore underwent UPPP. Snoring and apneas can be simulated by most people, and a direct effect of the Mueller maneuver may be seen during wakefulness. Thus, snoring simulation and the effects of the Mueller maneuver have been used in upper airway evaluation before surgical intervention in patients to predict surgical outcome and to improve patient selection.

CEPHALOMETRIC RADIOGRAPHY

Radiographic cephalometry has provided substantial insights into the pathophysiology of OSA (**Fig. 3**), demonstrating significant craniofacial characteristics associated with this disease. Although the results are not easy to compare,

Table 1			
Upper airway anatomy classification of Mueller's maneuver			
	Site of Obstruction	**Oropharynx**	**Hypopharynx**
Type 1 N(+,-)	Normal palatal position oropharyngeal	3+, 4+	0, 1+
Type 2 N(+,-)	Low palatal position	3+, 4+	1+, 2+
	a. predominantly oropharynx	3+, 4+	3+, 4+
	b. oro-hypopharynx involved		
Type 3	Normal orophayrnx–hypopharyngeal obstruction (retrognathia, micrognatia)	0, 1+	3+, 4+

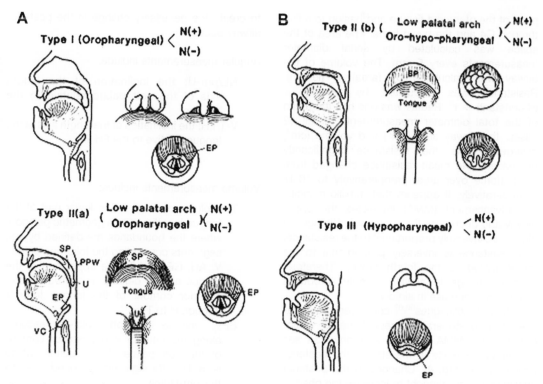

Fig. 2. The degree of pharyngeal obstruction at each level is determined by the reduction of pharyngeal lumen and is recorded as: 0, no collapse; 1+, 25% reduction of cross-sectional area; 2+, 50% reduction in area; 3+, 75% reduction in area; 4+, for complete obstruction (A, B).

specific cephalometric characteristics have been mentioned repeatedly as risk factors for OSA (eg, a thick and long soft palate, a retroposition of the maxilla or mandible, and especially the more inferiorly positioned hyoid bone).

Cephalometric evaluation provides a simple, inexpensive, readily accessible, and valuable method of screening. It provides longitudinal comparison over time and populations.[63] It is also useful for measuring airway changes in patients before and after treatment. Cephalometric analysis is readily available by OMS and orthodontists. Cephalometric studies have shown that patients who have OSAS have a shorter cranial base and a smaller cranial base flexure angle. Sleep apnea patients frequently have a cranial base length of 76.5 mm (normal, 83.3 mm) and a cranial base flexure angle of 122° (normal, 129°).[28,64]

Waite and Shettar reported a study[65] of 42 patients with OSAS. All patients were evaluated for the purpose of correlating surgical advancement with change in posterior airway space area, volume, and resistance. Cephalometrics were obtained preoperatively, immediately postoperatively, and at least 1 month later. The length of the airway space was defined from the lowest

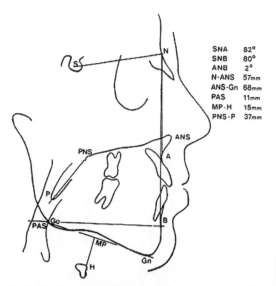

Fig. 3. Cephalometric analysis (normal values): S, sella; N, nasion; A, subspinale; B, supramentale; ANS, anterior nasal spine; PNS, posterior nasal spine; Go, gonion; Gn, gnathion; H, hyoid; PAS, posterior nasal spine; P, palate.

point of the pterygoid fissure and basion to a line through C4 and the hyoid bone. The area of the space was calculated by serial diameter measurements every 5 mm. The volume of the airway was calculated by (area) × (length). Resistance was calculated by (length) × (K constant) ÷ r^4. Radius was one half the mean of the total diameter measurements. In all 42 cases, the airway area (cm^2) and volume (cm^3) enlarged, while the resistance significantly decreased. The mean resistance changed from 28.72 (force over area) preoperatively to 10.47 postoperatively. It appears that maxillo-mandibular-advancement (MMA) increases the upper airway and decreases the resistance. Changes in airflow are inversely proportional to the resistance, and resistance is inversely proportional to the radius raised to the fourth power. Therefore, a small change in airway diameter produces a significant increase in airflow.

Waite and colleagues[66,67] compared preoperative and postoperative cephalometric radiographs after MMA surgery, and one can see a dramatic increase in the size of the posterior airway space (**Fig. 4**). Changes in the posterior airway space are thought to increase the pharyngeal volume and decrease the airway resistance. Cephalometric radiographs, however, are not the best method for evaluating the pharyngeal air space. There are patients with severe apnea who appear to have normal cephalometric analysis and adequate posterior airway spaces. The limitations of cephalometry are that it is only two-dimensional and not dynamic. It is not yet possible to calculate the amount of MMA needed to create the necessary change in the posterior airway space.

Angular measurements include:

NL/pm-U: the inclination of the length axis of the soft palate relative to the NL line

V-T/FH: the inclination of the length axis of the tongue relative to the FH line

Volume measurements include:

TV: volume of tongue. The lower part of the tongue is reduced to a geometric polygon, where the boundaries are defined by line segments connecting the following points: V, AH, GE, and T. The upper part of the tongue area is defined as the dorsal and superior contour of the tongue from V through H to T

SPV: volume of soft palate—measures along the anterior and posterior contour of the soft palate. The superior outline is a line through pm perpendicular to the pm-U-line

OV: oral volume—includes tongue volume and extends superiorly to the outline of the soft and hard palate

OPV: oropharyngeal volume—includes OV and the area defined by the point pm, upper pharyngeal wall, lower pharyngeal wall, and V along the posterior pharyngeal wall and the dorsal outline of the tongue, including the SPV

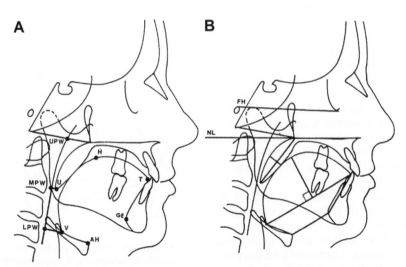

Fig. 4. (A) Depicts the landmarks of pharyngeal airway. (B) Demonstrates the linear measurements of the pharyngeal airway. (*Data from* Lyberg T, Krogstad O, Djupesland G. Cephalometric analysis in patients with obstructive sleep apnoea syndrome: II. Soft tissue morphology. J Laryngol Otol 1989;103(3):293–97.)

Ratios include:

TV/OV: relation between the tongue and oral volume

TV/OPV: relationship between tongue and the oropharyngeal volume

SPV/OV: relation between the soft palate and oral volume

SPV/OPV: relationship between soft palate and the oropharyngeal volume

CT

CT scanning significantly improves soft tissue contrast and allows precise measurements of cross-sectional areas at different levels and three dimensional reconstruction and volumetric assessment. Li and colleagues[44] stated the value of three-dimensional CT scan in providing the surgeon with anatomic information relevant in planning the upper airway surgery and monitoring its outcome. The geometry and caliber of the upper airway in apneic patients differ from those in normal subjects.[68] The apneic airway is smaller and is narrowed laterally. The volume of upper airway changed mildly between 9.2 cm^3 and 11.56 cm^3 in expiration and inspiration phases in a normal individual while sleeping. It fluctuated moderately between 3.74 cm^3 and 9.91 cm^3 in a habitual snorer, and changed acutely between 2.73 cm^3 and 16.01 cm^3 in an OSAS patient. Anatomic abnormalities of the pharynx are thought to play a role in the pathogenesis of OSAS49. The retropalatal space is the most relevant upper airway three-dimensional CT scan parameter identified in sleep-disordered breathing patients, and it is significantly associated with a compromised airway caliber.[44] This is thought to be one of the reasons for the decrease in apnea-hypo-nea-index (AHI) found during postoperative poly-somnographic studies.

During jaw surgery, the muscles, ligaments, and tendons are not detached but passively tightened with the advancement of their bony origins. This results in a modification of pharyngeal and palatal muscles, and the lingual and suprahyoid muscles. With skeletal expansion, there is enlargement of the pharyngeal soft tissue tube. The effectiveness of MMA is most likely a combination of a change in tension in the suprahyoid and velopharyngeal muscles, and the mechanical enlargement of the posterior airway space. Advancement of the maxilla pulls the soft tissue of the palate forward and upward. It also pulls the palatoglossal muscles forward and increases tongue support. Waite and colleagues[67] found that MMA enlarges the entire velopharynx by elevating the tissues attached to the maxilla, mandible, and hyoid, and results in increased tension on suprahyoid and velopharyngeal musculature (**Figs. 5** and **6**). Their study showed airway enhancement in the anteroposterior and lateral dimensions. Subsequently, investigations have begun to evaluate the changes in the poste-rior airway space by three-dimensional MRI.[68] Again, it appears that advancement of the tongue and widening of the lateral pillars occur with mandibular advancement.

MRI

Compared with lateral radiographic cephalometry or CT scanning, MRI offers various advantages, such as excellent soft tissue contrast, three-dimensional assessments of tissue structures, and lack of ionized radiation. The advantages with regard to the lack of ionized radiation have made MRI the imaging technique of choice for as-sessing children with SDB (sleep-disordered breathing). Schwab and colleagus[68] used MRI to study the upper airway and surrounding soft tissue structures in 21 normal subjects, 21 snorer/mild apneic subjects, and 26 patients with OSAS. They reported that at minimum airway area, thick-ness of the lateral pharyngeal muscular walls, rather than enlargement of the parapharyngeal fat pads, was the predominant anatomic factor causing airway narrowing in patients who had sleep apnea. The fat pad size at the level of the minimum airway was not greater in apneic than normal subjects. Shintani and colleagues[51] sug-gested dynamic MRI is useful to detect the level of occlusion during sleep and the severity of OSAS, and this can assist in treatment. In addition, they found the severity of AHI and oxygen satura-tion (SpO2) is correlated significantly with the width of the airway space at the base of the tongue and hypopharynx. By statistic pressure area rela-tionships, Isono and colleagues[30] found that the passive pharynx is more narrow and collapsible in sleep apnea patients than in matched controls. This is consistent with the other studies.[51,69] The retropositioned mandible will allow the tongue to impinge on the pharyngeal airway and decrease the air flow during sleep. The severity of AHI and SpO2 is correlated significantly with the width of the airway space at the base of the tongue and hypopharynx.[51] Ultrafast MRI is a reliable noninva-sive method for use in the evaluation of OSA.[70] The significant correlation between the findings at dynamic MRI and those at transnasal fiberoptic endoscopy shows that it is possible to detect the site of pharyngeal narrowing and occlusion with functional ultrafast MRI in awake patients.

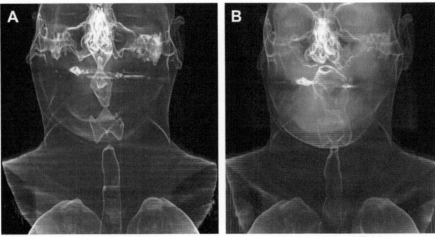

Pre-operative MMA   Postoperative MMA

Fig. 5. Pre- (*A*) and postoperative (*B*) front-view MMA images of the OSAS patient with subtraction three-dimensional CT scan demonstrate lateral enhancement of the airway.

ECHO IMAGING, ACOUSTIC REFLECTION TECHNOLOGY

Acoustic reflection provides a means to assess the patient's airway. It emits sound waves through a self-contained central processing unit comprised of two tools: the rhinometer and pharyngometer. They map the patient's nasal passages and pharyngeal airway, respectively. Acoustic reflection is a noninvasive technique based on the analysis of a sound wave reflected from the respiratory system. Acoustic reflectance permits the calculation of upper airway area as a function of distance from the mouth. Acoustic reflection does not provide anatomic information on discrete structures. Upper airway area calculations obtained with acoustic reflection therefore may not compare with other imaging modalities, in which the mouth remains closed during imaging. Acoustic reflection has been used for the comparative assessment of pharynx size among snorers, nonsnorers, and patients with OSAS.[71–73] It has the advantage of being noninvasive and quick, and it also allows for continuous evaluation of the patency of these regions. The technique, however, has two major restrictions; it cannot be used during sleep, and it cannot assess the nasopharynx.

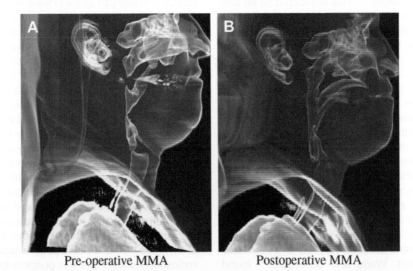

Pre-operative MMA   Postoperative MMA

Fig. 6. Pre- (*A*) and postoperative (*B*) side-view MMA images of the OSAS patient with subtraction three-dimensional CT scan demonstrate anteroposterior enhancement of the airway.

FLUOROSCOPY

Fluoroscopy provides information about the dynamic function of the airway and the level of stenosis or occlusion during sleep. Tsushima and colleagues[74] stated digital fluoroscopy displays the dynamic changes of the upper airways throughout the respiratory cycle. The velopharynx is the area where upper airway collapse most often begins.[26,75–78] Oropharyngeal obstruction also may occur, usually promoted by increased negative inspiratory pressure after primary velopharyngeal obstruction. Dynamic fluoroscopic sleep studies are a useful adjunct to endoscopy for evaluating OSA.[79–81] In children, the findings obtained from dynamic sleep fluoroscopy performed with sedation have been shown to affect treatment decisions in more than 50% of patients.[79] Only transverse images, however, can be obtained, in spite of the complex anatomy of the upper airway. The partial volume effect may affect the measurement of airway size. Digital fluoroscopy provides only a two-dimensional lateral view, so that only the anterior–posterior dimensions can be appreciated. In apnea patients, the airway has an anterior–posterior configuration unlike normal subjects, who had a horizontal configuration with the major axis in the lateral direction. This change of the upper airway shape cannot be shown from the lateral view of digital fluoroscopy. The lateral dimension of the upper airway may be as important as the anteroposterior dimension.

CFD

In addition to simple two-dimensional assessment, researchers have begun to evaluate volumes of soft tissue structures such as the tongue, the adenoids, the soft palate, the pharyngeal walls, and the remaining compromised or noncompromised airway spaces. To obtain three-dimensional data, volumes are calculated on cross-sectional areas, and slice thickness is established by various computerized models. After several decades of computer development, computer-aided engineering (CAE) has become a matured technology that plays an important role in the engineering community for design, analyses, and performance predictions.[82,83] The development has become especially significant during the past two decades, when computer hardware performance–cost ratio has increased. This provides the computational engineers with computing resources that were unimaginable just a decade ago. The enabling technologies associated with CAE involve the scientific disciplines of numerical geometry modeling, numerical mesh generation, scientific visualization, virtual environment technology, and high-performance parallel computing. They enable simulation disciplines such as CFD and computational structure mechanics (CSM), which use numerical methods to solve the governing equations that provide high-fidelity computational simulations of fluid flow transport phenomena and structure behaviors.[84] Such computational technologies can benefit the medical communities in understanding airflow and hemodynamics of human biologic systems.[83,85]

To enable these computational technologies, the first step is to generate high-quality numerical meshes while maintaining geometry fidelity from CT imaging. There have been many numerical geometry algorithms presented during the past few decades, such as the cubic spline, Hermit spline, Bezier spline, and B-spline.[86] Among them, the nonuniform rational B-spline (NURBS, **Fig. 7**) has gained great popularity in the CAE community and is the de facto industry standard for the representation and design of a geometry algorithms.[87]

AIRFLOW MODELING FOR OSAS
Steps Involved in the Modeling

The high-fidelity three-dimensional numerical analyses have not yet been performed to understand the dynamics of the airflow in the human airway for surgical treatment of OSAS. To enable these computational technologies, the first step is to generate high-quality numerical meshes while maintaining geometric fidelity. Mesh generation is a step preceding computational simulations. It is very crucial to have high-quality meshes, as the quality of meshes plays an essential role in the numerical simulations and affects the computational efficiency in terms of convergence and accuracy.[88]

Geometry generation: reconstruction of facial and airway geometry from three-dimensional CT scan

This preprocessing step is a critical step in numerical simulations, as the geometric fidelity and mesh quality can greatly affect both the convergence of numerical calculations, and more importantly, the accuracy of the result.

When a CT image dataset is acquired, there can be many factors[89,90] that affect its quality other than the resolution. The noise in the dataset is one of the issues that must be addressed. This issue can be mitigated through the use of mathematical algorithms. With a view to the desire to use the image data for segmentation and surface

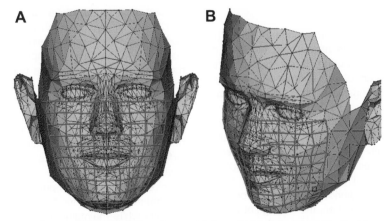

Fig. 7. (*A*) A NURBS surface and (*B*) a NURBS surface patch is mapped onto a hypothetical human face, and the control point new location can be calculated based on the surface perturbation.

extraction, one can remove noise selectively through the careful application of selected three-dimensional imaging mathematical filters. It is important to keep the use of such filtering to an absolute minimum, so that the resulting image is as coherent to the original as possible, while attempting to remove only noise and other unneeded information. The authors found that using a three-dimensional median convolution filter followed by three-dimensional Gaussian blur filter removes most undesirable noise while still maintaining a high fidelity to the original image. To extract the desired geometry of the airway, the three-dimensional image data must be segmented. Surfaces defined by a radical shift in the scalar values in the image volume are relatively simple to segment. Examples of these types of surfaces include bone boundaries in CT data and the boundary between flesh and air in CT or MRI data. This process, however, will require the research team members from both the medical and engineering communities to work closely to make sure that proper surface information is extracted. The National Library of Medicine Insight Segmentation and Registration Toolkit[91] (ITK, www.itk.org) provides many advanced noise reduction and segmentation algorithms that will be leveraged with for this work **Fig. 8** shows the area of interest and the preliminary effort to extract the boundary surfaces of the geometry of interest. This example indicates the appropriate approaches as suggested. More efforts, however, are needed to enhance the algorithms to extract the geometry more accurately.

Generation of numerical meshes
Once the geometry of interest is extracted, numerical meshes must be generated before CFD simulations can take place. This requires the numerical mesh generation algorithms to be robust for complex biologic geometry to generate quality meshes suitable for CFD simulations. **Fig. 2**

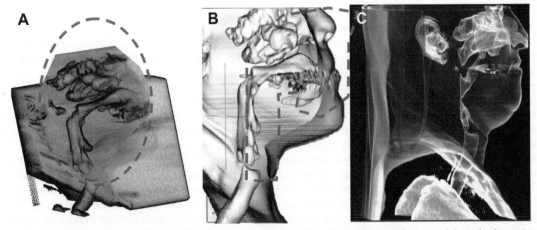

Fig. 8. Preliminary result of volume rendering (*A*), extracting surfaces for geometry of interest (*B*), and subtraction three-dimensional CT scan (*C*).

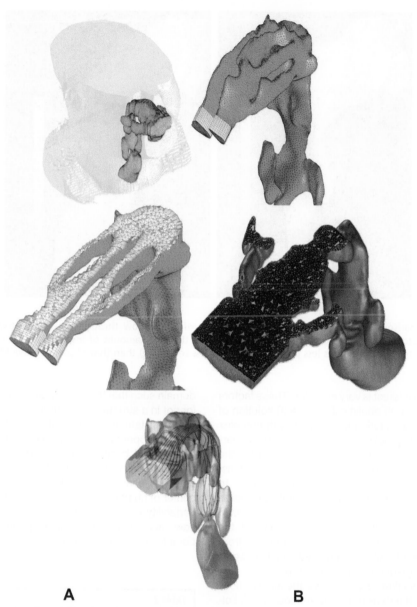

A   **B**

Fig. 9. Geometry and mesh for the preoperative MMA. (*A*) Surface mesh with extensions needed for CFD simulations (*yellow*). (*B*) Cross section of the hybrid mesh.

illustrates a mesh generated by a modified decimation method for surface meshes[92] and a hybrid mesh generation method.[93] These methods were developed at the enabling technology laboratory, and create high-quality meshes consistently. **Fig. 9** shows the cutaway view of the hybrid mesh, which is a combination of prismatic meshes for the region near the wall and tetrahedral meshes for the rest of the domain. Such meshes will be used for simulations of flow fields using sophisticated computational fluid dynamics (CFD) software developed at computational simulation lab.

CFD visualization

The geometry of the upper airway is extracted, and the associated mesh is generated. CFD-based numerical simulations can be performed to analyze the transport phenomena of flow through the airway. The CFD-based numerical simulation is conducted by solving the governing equations, which describe the transport phenomena of continuum fluid flows such as air. The governing equation consists of a set of coupled nonlinear equations (continuity, momentum, and energy equations[84]), and the

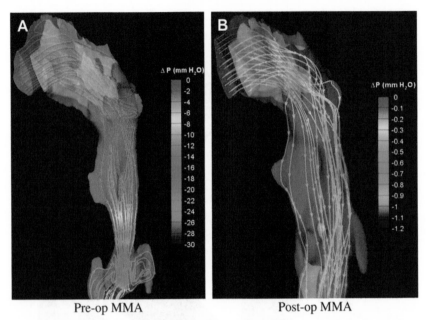

Pre-op MMA   Post-op MMA

Fig. 10. Comparison of streamlines and pressures efforts of the airflow through the upper airway between pre- and postoperative MMA using CFD simulations. With the same amount of inspired air, the upper airway of postoperative MMA requires less pressure effort (ie, less resistance) than that of preoperative MMA.

geometry of interest is very complex. These factors make deriving an analytical (ie, exact) solution of the governing equation for the flow with complex geometries impractical. Hence, numerous numerical methods have been developed to solve the set of coupled nonlinear governing equations. There are two major approaches employed to solve the governing equations: pressure-based and density-based methods. The pressure-based method, which solves pressure as one of the dependent variables and obtains density from the equation of state, is employed widely to solve the low-to-medium speed incompressible and compressible flow, especially for the internal flow. In contrast, the density-based method, which solves density as one of the dependent variables and obtains pressure from the equation of state, most often is used to solve the compressible high-speed flow, especially for the external flow. Each method has its strengths and weaknesses. In terms of grid topology, there are two major approaches used in CFD solvers: structured grid and unstructured grid solvers. The structured grid flow solvers employ either quadrilateral (for two-dimensional) or hexahedral (for three-dimensional) mesh to discretize the flow domain of interest, such that indices of the mesh are in order. The unstructured grid flow solvers use quadrilateral and triangular (for two-dimensional), or tetrahedral, hexahedral, prism, and pyramid (for three-dimensional) mesh to represent the computational

domain such that the mesh indices are not in order (or not in a structured manner).

To facilitate the CFD simulations of airway, pre- and postoperative airway geometries must be constructed based on the CT data, followed by numerical mesh generation to represent the discretized geometry (**Fig. 10**). The CFD flow solvers, center of numerical simulations, need to equip the capability of solving the low-speed compressible flow accurately and handling problems with complex geometries efficiently.

Table 2
The pressure efforts were decreased in all level of the airway after MMA

Level of the Airway	Pressure Effort (mm H$_2$O)	
	Preoperatively	Postoperatively
L1	−14.1	−0.34
L2	−13.38	−0.29
L3 (base of tongue)	−18.78	−0.35
L4	−7.52	−0.39
L5	−1.54	−0.32
L6	−0.72	−0.23
L7	−0.51	−0.04
L8	0	0

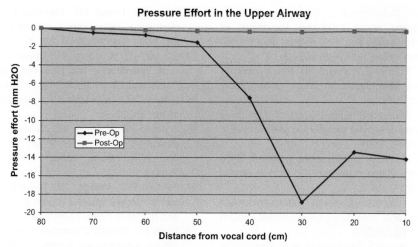

Fig. 11. The pressure efforts were decreased in all different levels of the airway after MMA.

After MMA, the CFD model shows less pressure efforts in all levels of the airway (**Table 2, Fig. 11**). It can be seen that the pressure effort decreases as the airway dimension (diameter and volume) increases. At the narrowest part of the airway (vocal cord), one can see the airflow has the highest value of pressure effort. The increase of the airway volume is a response to MMA surgery, and the region around the base of tongue has the most increase. MMA surgery helps the sleep apnea patients to breathe easier with less effort to breathe. It means these patients use less pressure effort to inhale the same amount of air compared with the effort measured in preoperative OSAS. In another words, these patients now use less energy to take a breath and do not need continuous positive airway pressure (CPAP). After MMA surgery, the AHI has been decreased from 28 to 5.8, and the airway volume has increased.

SUMMARY

The CFD simulations are conducted to obtain the pressure effort of the airflow through various pre- and postoperative geometries of upper airway. If one can prove in multiple subjects that all parameters of the airway (ie, pressure effort (ΔP), volume, and diameter of airway) at the relevant level (retro-palatal and retro-ligual areas), have correlations with clinical study parameters (BMI and polysomnogram such as AHI and SpO2), one should be able to define the correlation of the parameters in a mathematic formula with clinical relevance.

As with all treatment of disease, one must start with the correct diagnosis. Medical or dental imaging is an obvious benefit for prescribing the proper treatment intervention. OSAS is thought to be caused by obstruction of the upper airway,

with other variables such as neuromuscular reflex control, soft tissue abnormality, and poor skeletal support contributing. The exact site of collapse during sleep, however, is unknown. Surgeons try to direct intervention toward the most obvious site of obstruction using assumed case based protocols. There are no simple diagnostic tests to determine the location of obstruction and help prescribe or quantify the surgical intervention. A technique to a priori determine the success of an intervention or the amount of treatment therefore would be of great benefit. Fortunately, dynamic and accurate imaging of the upper airway is available, which will allow patient-specific treatment based upon anatomic variation. The most recently developed techniques that provide such realistic promise consist of the biomedical application of computational fluid dynamics or CFD.

REFERENCES

1. Young T, Palta M, Dempsey J, et al. The occurrence of sleep-disordered breathing among middle-aged adults. N Engl J Med 1993;328(17):1230–5.
2. Young T, Peppard PE, Gottlieb DJ. Epidemiology of obstructive sleep apnea: a population health perspective. Am J Respir Crit Care Med 2002; 165(9):1217–39.
3. Guilleminault C, Tilkian A, Dement WC. The sleep apnea syndromes. Annu Rev Med 1976;27:465–84.
4. Young T, Peppard P. Sleep-disordered breathing and cardiovascular disease: epidemiologic evidence for a relationship. Sleep 2000;23(Suppl 4): S122–6.
5. Young T, Peppard P, Palta M, et al. Population-based study of sleep-disordered breathing as a risk factor for hypertension. Arch Intern Med 1997;157(15): 1746–52.

6. Tilkian AG, Guilleminault C, Schroeder JS, et al. Sleep-induced apnea syndrome. Prevalence of cardiac arrhythmias and their reversal after tracheostomy. Am J Med 1977;63(3):348–58.

7. Young T, Skatrud J, Peppard PE. Risk factors for obstructive sleep apnea in adults. JAMA 2004; 291(16):2013–6.

8. Young T, Peppard P. Epidemiology of obstructive sleep apnea. Breathing disorders in sleep. London: W.B. Saunders; 2001.

9. Maekawa M, Shiomi T. Sleep apnea syndrome (SAS) and ischemic heart disease (IHD). Nippon Rinsho 2000;58(8):1702–6.

10. Chin K. Obstructive sleep apnea–hypopnea syndrome and cardiovascular diseases. Intern Med 2004;43(7):527–8.

11. Beelke M, Angeli S, Del Sette M, et al. Obstructive sleep apnea can be provocative for right-to-left shunting through a patent foramen ovale. Sleep 2002;25(8):856–62.

12. Altin R, Ozdemir H, Mahmutyazicioglu K, et al. Evaluation of carotid artery wall thickness with high-resolution sonography in obstructive sleep apnea syndrome. J Clin Ultrasound 2005;33(2):80–6.

13. George CF. Sleep. 5: driving and automobile crashes in patients with obstructive sleep apnoea/hypopnoea syndrome. Thorax 2004;59(9):804–7.

14. George CF, Smiley A. Sleep apnea & automobile crashes. Sleep 1999;22(6):790–5.

15. Wu H, Yan-Go F. Self-reported automobile accidents involving patients with obstructive sleep apnea. Neurology 1996;46(5):1254–7.

16. Krieger J, McNicholas WT, Levy P, et al. Public health and medico-legal implications of sleep apnoea. Eur Respir J 2002;20(6):1594–609.

17. Strollo PJ Jr, Rogers RM. Obstructive sleep apnea. N Engl J Med 1996;334(2):99–104.

18. Sher AE. Surgical management of obstructive sleep apnea. Prog Cardiovasc Dis 1999;41(5): 387–96.

19. Peter JH, Becker H, Cassel W, et al. Diagnosis of sleep apnea: initial experiences with a staged procedure. Pneumologie 1989;43(Suppl 1):587–90.

20. Conradt R, Hochban W, Brandenburg U, et al. Long-term follow-up after surgical treatment of obstructive sleep apnoea by maxillomandibular advancement. Eur Respir J 1997;10(1):123–8.

21. Nimkarn Y, Miles PG, Waite PD. Maxillomandibular advancement surgery in obstructive sleep apnea syndrome patients: long-term surgical stability. J Oral Maxillofac Surg 1995;53(12):1414–8 [discussion: 1418–9].

22. Pepin JL, Ferretti G, Veale D, et al. Somnofluoroscopy, computed tomography, and cephalometry in the assessment of the airway in obstructive sleep apnoea. Thorax 1992;47(3):150–6.

23. Riley RW, Powell NB. Maxillofacial surgery and obstructive sleep apnea syndrome. Otolaryngol Clin North Am 1990;23(4):809–26.

24. Schwab RJ, Goldberg AN. Upper airway assessment: radiographic and other imaging techniques. Otolaryngol Clin North Am 1998;31(6):931–68.

25. Schwab RJ. Upper airway imaging. Clin Chest Med 1998;19(1):33–54.

26. Shepard JW Jr, Gefter WB, Guilleminault C, et al. Evaluation of the upper airway in patients with obstructive sleep apnea. Sleep 1991;14(4): 361–71.

27. Turnbull NR, Battagel JM. The effects of orthognathic surgery on pharyngeal airway dimensions and quality of sleep. J Orthod 2000;27(3):235–47.

28. Waite PD, Wooten V, Lachner J, et al. Maxillomandibular advancement surgery in 23 patients with obstructive sleep apnea syndrome. J Oral Maxillofac Surg 1989;47(12):1256–61 [discussion: 1262].

29. Isono S. Diagnosis of sites of upper airway obstruction in patients with obstructive sleep apnea. Nippon Rinsho 2000;58(8):1660–4.

30. Isono S, Feroah TR, Hajduk EA, et al. Interaction of cross-sectional area, driving pressure, and airflow of passive velopharynx. J Appl Phys 1997;83(3): 851–9.

31. Isono S, Morrison DL, Launois SH, et al. Static mechanics of the velopharynx of patients with obstructive sleep apnea. J Appl Phys 1993;75(1): 148–54.

32. Isono S, Remmers JE, Tanaka A, et al. Anatomy of pharynx in patients with obstructive sleep apnea and in normal subjects. J Appl Phys 1997;82(4): 1319–26.

33. Isono S, Shimada A, Utsugi M, et al. Comparison of static mechanical properties of the passive pharynx between normal children and children with sleep-disordered breathing. Am J Respir Crit Care Med 1998;157:1204–12.

34. Isono S, Tanaka A, Tagaito Y, et al. Pharyngeal patency in response to advancement of the mandible in obese anesthetized persons. Anesthesiology 1997;87(5):1055–62.

35. Launois SH, Feroah TR, Campbell WN, et al. Site of pharyngeal narrowing predicts outcome of surgery for obstructive sleep apnea. Am Rev Respir Dis 1993;147(1):182–9.

36. Morrison DL, Launois SH, Isono S, et al. Pharyngeal narrowing and closing pressures in patients with obstructive sleep apnea. Am Rev Respir Dis 1993; 148(3):606–11.

37. Saeki N, Isono S, Tanaka A, et al. Pre-and postoperative respiratory assessment of acromegalics with sleep apnea—bedside oximetric study for transsphenoidal approach. Endocrinol Jpn 2000;47: S61–4.

38. Watanabe T, Isono S, Tanaka A, et al. Contribution of body habitus and craniofacial characteristics to segmental closing pressures of the passive pharynx in patients with sleep-disordered breathing. Am J Respir Crit Care Med 2002;165(2):260–5.

39. Hsu PP, Tan BY, Chan YH, et al. Clinical predictors in obstructive sleep apnea patients with computer-assisted quantitative videoendoscopic upper airway analysis. Laryngoscope 2004;114(5): 791–9.

40. Abbott MB, Donnelly LF, Dardzinski BJ, et al. Obstructive sleep apnea: MR imaging volume segmentation analysis. Radiology 2004;232(3):889–95.

41. Adams GL, Gansky SA, Miller AJ, et al. Comparison between traditional 2-dimensional cephalometry and a 3-dimensional approach on human dry skulls. Am J Orthod Dentofacial Orthop 2004;126(4): 397–409.

42. Hoffman EA, Gefter WB. Multimodality imaging of the upper airway: MRI, MR spectroscopy, and ultrafast X-ray CT. Prog Clin Biol Res 1990;345: 291–301.

43. Joseph AA, Elbaum J, Cisneros GJ, et al. A cephalometric comparative study of the soft tissue airway dimensions in persons with hyperdivergent and normodivergent facial patterns. J Oral Maxillofac Surg 1998;56(2):135–9 [discussion: 139–40].

44. Li HY, Chen NH, Wang CR, et al. Use of 3-dimensional computed tomography scan to evaluate upper airway patency for patients undergoing sleep-disordered breathing surgery. Otolaryngol Head Neck Surg 2003;129(4):336–42.

45. Lowe AA, Gionhaku N, Takeuchi K, et al. Three-dimensional CT reconstructions of tongue and airway in adult subjects with obstructive sleep apnea. Am J Orthod Dentofacial Orthop 1986;90(5):364–74.

46. Lyberg T, Krogstad O, Djupesland G. Cephalometric analysis in patients with obstructive sleep apnoea syndrome: II. Soft tissue morphology. J Laryngol Otol 1989;103(3):293–7.

47. Metes A, Hoffstein V, Direnfeld V, et al. Three-dimensional CT reconstruction and volume measurements of the pharyngeal airway before and after maxillofacial surgery in obstructive sleep apnea. J Otolaryngol 1993;22(4):261–4.

48. Martonen TB, Zhang Z, Yu G, et al. Three-dimensional computer modeling of the human upper respiratory tract. Cell Biochem Biophys 2001;35(3):255–61.

49. Oda M, Suzuka Y, Lan Z, et al. Evaluation of pharyngolaryngeal region with 3-D computed tomography. Int Congr Ser 2003;1257:281–7.

50. Schwab RJ, Gefter WB, Hoffman EA, et al. Dynamic upper airway imaging during awake respiration in normal subjects and patients with sleep disordered breathing. Am Rev Respir Dis 1993;148(5): 1385–400.

51. Shintani T, Kozawa T, Himi T. Obstructive sleep apnea by analysis of MRI findings. Int Congr Ser 2003;1257:99–102.

52. Schwab RJ. Imaging for the snoring and sleep apnea patient. Dent Clin North Am 2001;45(4): 759–96.

53. Friedman M, Tanyeri H, La Rosa M, et al. Clinical predictors of obstructive sleep apnea. Laryngoscope 1999;109(12):1901–7.

54. Friedman M, Ibrahim H, Joseph NJ. Staging of obstructive sleep apnea/hypopnea syndrome: a guide to appropriate treatment. Laryngoscope 2004;114(3):454–9.

55. Friedman M, Vidyasagar R, Bliznikas D, et al. Does severity of obstructive sleep apnea/hypopnea syndrome predict uvulopalatopharyngoplasty outcome? Laryngoscope 2005;115(12): 2109–13.

56. Li HY, Wang PC, Lee LA, et al. Prediction of uvulopalatopharyngoplasty outcome: anatomy-based staging system versus severity-based staging system. Sleep 2006;29(12):1537–41.

57. Woodson BT. Examination of upper airway. Oral Maxillofac Surg Clin North Am 1995;7:257–67.

58. Katsantonis GP, Maas CS, Walsh JK. The predictive efficacy of the Muller maneuver in uvulopalatopharyngoplasty. Laryngoscope 1989;99:677–80.

59. Kuna ST, Bedi DG, Ryckman C. Effect of nasal airway positive pressure on upper airway size and configuration. Am Rev Respir Dis 1988;138(4): 969–75.

60. Lavie P, Fischel N, Zomer J, et al. The effects of partial and complete mechanical occlusion of the nasal passages on sleep structure and breathing in sleep. Acta Otolaryngol 1983;95:161–6.

61. Catalfumo FJ, Golz A, Westerman ST, et al. The epiglottis and obstructive sleep apnoea syndrome. J Laryngol Otol 1998;112(10):940–3.

62. Sher AE, Thorpy MJ, Shprintzen RJ, et al. Predictive value of Muller maneuver in selection of patients for uvulopalatopharyngoplasty. Laryngoscope 1985; 95(12):1483–7.

63. Hans MG, Goldberg J. Cephalometric exam in obstructive sleep apnea. Oral Maxillofac Surg Clin North Am 1995;7:209–81.

64. Steinberg B, Fraser B. The cranial base in obstructive sleep apnea. J Oral Maxillofac Surg 1995; 53(10):1150–4.

65. Waite PD, Shetter SM. Maxillomandibular advancement surgery: a cure for obstructive sleep apnea syndrome. Oral Maxillofac Surg Clin North Am 1995;7:327–36.

66. Waite PD. Obstructive sleep apnea: a review of the pathophysiology and surgical management. Oral Surg Oral Med Oral Pathol Oral Radiol Endod 1998;85(4):352–61.

67. Waite PD, Vilos GA. Surgical changes of posterior airway space in obstructive sleep apnea. Oral Maxillofac Surg Clin North Am 2002;14:385–99.

68. Schwab RJ, Gupta KB, Gefter WB, et al. Upper airway and soft tissue anatomy in normal subjects and patients with sleep-disordered breathing. Significance of the lateral pharyngeal walls. Am J Respir Crit Care Med 1995;152:1673–89.

69. Fouke JM, Wolin AD, Strohl KP, et al. Elastic characteristics of the airway wall. J Appl Phys 1989;66(2): 962–7.

70. Jager L, Gunther E, Gauger J, et al. Fluoroscopic MR of the pharynx in patients with obstructive sleep apnea. AJNR Am J Neuroradiol 1998;19(7): 1205–14.

71. Brooks LJ, Strohl KP. Size and mechanical properties of the pharynx in healthy men and women. Am Rev Respir Dis 1992;146(6):1394–7.

72. Brown IB, McClean PA, Boucher R, et al. Changes in pharyngeal cross-sectional area with posture and application of continuous positive airway pressure in patients with obstructive sleep apnea. Am Rev Respir Dis 1987;136(3):628–32.

73. Hoffstein V, Wright S, Zamel N, et al. Pharyngeal function and snoring characteristics in apneic and nonapneic snorers. Am Rev Respir Dis 1991; 143(6):1294–9.

74. Tsushima Y, Antila J, Svedstrom E, et al. Upper airway size and collapsibility in snorers: evaluation with digital fluoroscopy. Eur Respir J 1996;9(8): 1611–8.

75. Suratt PM, Dee P, Atkinson RL, et al. Fluoroscopic and computed tomographic features of the pharyngeal airway in obstructive sleep apnea. Am Rev Respir Dis 1983;127(4):487–92.

76. Hudgel DW. Variable site of airway narrowing among obstructive sleep apnea patients. J Appl Phys 1986; 61(4):1403–9.

77. Hudgel DW, Hendricks C. Palate and hypopharynx—sites of inspiratory narrowing of the upper airway during sleep. Am Rev Respir Dis 1988; 138(6):1542–7.

78. Katsantonis GP, Walsh JK. Somnofluoroscopy: its role in the selection of candidates for uvulopalatopharyngoplasty. Otolaryngol Head Neck Surg 1986;94(1):56–60.

79. Gibson SE, Myer CM 3rd, Strife JL, et al. Sleep fluoroscopy for localization of upper airway obstruction in children. Ann Otol Rhinol Laryngol 1996;105(9):678–83.

80. Donnelly LF, Strife JL, Myer CM 3rd. Is sedation safe during dynamic sleep fluoroscopy of children with obstructive sleep apnea? AJR Am J Roentgenol 2001;177(5):1031–4.

81. Donnelly LF, Strife JL, Myer CM 3rd. Glossoptosis (posterior displacement of the tongue) during sleep: a frequent cause of sleep apnea in pediatric patients referred for dynamic sleep fluoroscopy. AJR Am J Roentgenol 2000;175(6):1557–60.

82. Sharit J. Perspectives on computer aiding in cognitive work domains: toward predictions of effectiveness and use. Ergonomics 2003;46:126–40.

83. Gore BF. Human performance cognitive-behavioral modeling: a benefit for occupational safety. Int J Occup Saf Ergon 2002;8(3):339–51.

84. Warsi ZUA. Fluid dynamics: theoretical and computational approaches. 3rd edition. CRC Press, Incorporated; 1998.

85. Wong BK, Sellaro CL, Monaco JA. Information systems analysis approach in hospitals: a national survey. Health Care Superv 1995;13(3):58–64.

86. Farin GE. Curves and surfaces for CAGD: a practical guide. 5th edition. Morgan Kaufmann; 2001.

87. Piegl LA, Tiller W. The NURBS book. 2nd edition. Springer Verlag; 1997.

88. Thompson JF, Warsi ZUA, Mastin CW. Numerical grid generation: foundations and applications. New York: Elsevier North-Holland, Incorporated; 1985.

89. Russ JC. The image processing handbook. 2nd edition. Boca Raton (FL): CRC Press; 1995.

90. Kuwahara M. Processing of RI-angiocardiographic images, in digital processing of biomedical images. New York: Plenum Press; 1976.

91. Ibanez L, Schroeder W, Ng L, et al. ITK software guide. Kitware Incorporated; 2003.

92. Ito Y, Shum PC, Shih AM, et al. Robust generation of high-quality unstructured meshes on realistic biomedical geometry. Int J Numer Methods Eng 2006;65(6):943–73.

93. Ito Y, Shih AM, Soni BK, et al. An approach to generate high-quality unstructured hybrid meshes. Presented at the 44th AIAA Aerospace Sciences Meeting and Exhibit. Reno (NV), 2006.

Management of Obstructive Sleep Apnea by Continuous Positive Airway Pressure

Terri E. Weaver, PhD, RN, FAAN*, Amy Sawyer, PhD, RN

KEYWORDS

- Continuous positive airway pressure
- CPAP • Adherence • Compliance
- Medical management • Obstructive sleep apnea

Obstructive sleep apnea (OSA) is a common problem, with 9% to 28% of women and 24% to 26% of males having apneic events at a treatable level, making this syndrome a serious public health issue.[1] Obstructive events occur when the upper pharyngeal walls repeatedly close during sleep, creating apneic and hypopneic events resulting in intermittent nocturnal hypoxia and sleep fragmentation.[2] The amount of pressure required to maintain airway patency is determined during a sleep study (titration polysomnography, PSG) where the pressure is titrated to eliminate apneas and hypopneas, as determined by a reduction in the apnea-hypopnea index (AHI, number of apneas and hypopneas per hour of sleep) and restore sleep architecture. The titration is performed during the entire PSG or conducted in the last half following a diagnostic first half (split-night study). Half of the 18 million Americans who suffer from OSA[3] are exposed to increased risk for significant morbidity and mortality, including increased cardiovascular risk,[1,4–7] insulin resistance,[7,8] systemic inflammation,[7] metabolic syndrome,[7] daytime sleepiness,[1,9] and automobile crashes[10–13] because they are nonadherent to the primary and most effective treatment for this syndrome, nasal continuous positive airway

pressure (CPAP).[14,15] CPAP eradicates the nocturnal upper pharyngeal closures, reversing the daytime impairments associated with OSA, Yet, the overall effectiveness of CPAP treatment is significantly limited by poor adherence and/or suboptimal use by many OSA patients.[9] This article describes the outcomes associated with CPAP treatment, significance of the issue of poor adherence in OSA, discusses evidence regarding the optimal duration of nightly use, describes the nature and predictors of nonadherence, and reviews interventions that have been tested to increase nightly use and suggests management strategies.

DOES CPAP MAKE A DIFFERENCE?

Although we would like to think that CPAP is the "magic bullet," there is mixed evidence regarding its effectiveness to improve neurobehavior, reduce cardiovascular disease, and alter insulin resistance, especially those with milder apnea.[16–18] The reduction in daytime sleepiness associated with CPAP treatment, often after one night's use with increased benefit up to 6 weeks,[16,18,19] led the American Academy of Sleep Medicine (Academy) to recommend this therapy as a standard indication for improving

Funding: Grant funding received from Cephalon, Inc.

Dr Weaver is a consultant for Cephalon, Inc and receives a royalty fee for the Functional Outcomes of Sleep Questionnaire from Philips Respironics.

Biobehavioral and Health Sciences Division, University of Pennsylvania School of Nursing, Claire M. Fagin Hall, 418 Curie Boulevard, Philadelphia, PA 19104-4217, USA

* Corresponding author.

E-mail address: tew@nursing.upenn.edu (T.E. Weaver).

self-reported sleepiness.[17] However, the resolution of daytime sleepiness is more profound in those with an AHI greater than 30. The ability to more fully engage in daily activities accompanies the decrease in daytime sleepiness associated with CPAP treatment.[9,16] Use of CPAP to improve the quality of life of OSA patients was recommended by the Academy only as a treatment option given the increased need for evidence from large controlled clinical trials.

Evaluating the evidence of the effectiveness of CPAP treatment on the cognitive and performance impairments exhibited by OSA patients is challenging because of differences across studies with regard to treatment adherence as well as study design issues including sample size, types of control populations, and the nature of placebos when they were used. Response to CPAP is more clearly demonstrated when comparisons are made only in those who manifest deficits in cognitive processing and performance at baseline and in those more adherent (eg, use of CPAP for 6 or more hours per night).[20] Indeed, improvements in cognitive and neurobehavioral performance may be a function of baseline level of daytime sleepiness.[21] When sham-CPAP was used as a control to examine treatment response in patients without subjective daytime sleepiness,[22] CPAP was not found to be superior to placebo with regard to cognitive outcomes. Further, in other placebo-controlled studies, mostly conducted in patients with moderate to severe OSA, the superiority of CPAP over placebo has not been demonstrated for cognitive functioning, sustained attention, or executive function.[16,21]

Whether CPAP improves blood pressure has been the largest area of investigation regarding cardiovascular treatment outcomes. Several meta-analyses involving large numbers of OSA participants have shown decreases in mean arterial pressure from −1.39 to 2.22 mm Hg, decrease in systolic blood pressure from −1.38 to 2.46 mm HG, and reduction in diastolic blood pressure from −1.48 to 1.83 mm HG.[23–25] In two of the three meta-analyses, these reductions, although small, were statistically significant and viewed as clinically important.[24,25] Moreover, a large study involving participants with mild to moderate sleep apnea demonstrated that CPAP treatment was associated with a cardiovascular risk reduction of 64% independent of age and preexisting cardiovascular comorbidities.[26] Collectively, these findings were the basis for the recommendation by the Academy that as a treatment option CPAP should be considered adjunctive therapy to lower blood pressure in hypertensive patients with OSA.[17] Studies that have examined the efficacy of CPAP to improve insulin resistance have provided conflicting results.[27–34] These inconsistencies may be related to characteristics of the study population, such as whether the study was conducted in obese OSA patients or in those with diabetes in addition to how insulin resistance was evaluated, sample size, and whether a control was used. Some studies have found improvements in glycosylated hemoglobin-a form of hemoglobin used to characterize average plasma glucose concentration (HbA_{1C}),[8,27] whereas others have found changes in metrics of insulin resistance, such as homeostatic model assessment, is a method used to quantify insulin (HOMA-β)[28] and sleeping and nocturnal glucose levels,[29] as well as insulin sensitivity.[31]

A major drawback in clinical trials to the successful evaluation of the efficacy of CPAP treatment across outcomes has been suboptimal adherence. Stradling and Davies[35] demonstrated a relationship between nightly hours of CPAP use and ratings of self-reported daytime sleepiness and Weaver and colleagues[9] showed that recovery of objectively and subjectively evaluated daytime sleepiness as well as functional status was affected by hours of nightly application of the device. Degree of CPAP adherence also determined recovery of normal neurobehavior performance in impaired OSA patients.[20] The important influence of treatment adherence in studies examining the impact of CPAP on cardiovascular disease is illustrated by the fact that although 24-hour mean blood pressure would have further decreased by 0.89 mm Hg if the sample had greater disease severity (10-point increase in AHI) ($P = .006$), that effect on blood pressure is even more profound when degree of adherence is considered.[24] Each 1-hour increase in effective nightly CPAP use by study participants would have resulted in a further reduction in 24-hour mean blood pressures of 1.39 mm Hg ($P = .01$).[24] Steiropoulos and colleagues[27] also found that changes in HbA_1 level following treatment occurred only in those applying the device more than 4 hours/night and Babu and co-investigators[8] found that only in those using CPAP more than 4 hours/night was the reduction in HbA_1 level correlated with days of CPAP use. With a mean nightly CPAP use of 4.46 hours across placebo-controlled randomized clinical trials in the extant literature,[16] it is possible that positive effects of CPAP treatment may have been unsupported because of reduced power associated with insufficient exposure, ie, adherence, to the intervention.

HOW SIGNIFICANT IS THE PROBLEM OF POOR ADHERENCE TO CPAP?

Despite the efficacy of CPAP in reversing sleep apnea, defining adequate nightly use of at least 4 hours per night, 29% to 83% of patients are non-adherent.[16,36–47] Sixteen years after this level of nonadherence was first described,[37] the pattern of CPAP adherence remains unchanged.[48,49] Although the average daily use of those who are adherent to CPAP is approximately 6 hours, those who routinely skip nights of use average only about 3 hours.[48] In other words, patients who are not adherent to CPAP not only fail to use it on many nights, but even when they apply it, the nightly duration of use is shorter than that of patients who are adherent. Although most CPAP users apply CPAP for the same duration on the first night of treatment, nonadherent users begin skipping nights of treatment in the first week of treatment.[48–51] By the second to fourth day of treatment, their hourly use of CPAP is significantly shorter than those who apply CPAP, suggesting early treatment or possibly pretreatment factors influence decisions to use CPAP.[48–51] More alarming is that patients who become nonadherent in the first few days of CPAP treatment generally remain nonadherent.[48,49,52,53] The return of symptoms and other manifestations of OSA with nonuse of CPAP, even for one night, underscores the need for adherence to treatment to realize positive physiological and behavioral outcomes.[54,55]

WHAT CPAP "DOSE" RESULTS IN IMPROVED HEALTH AND FUNCTIONAL OUTCOMES?

There have been several studies that have attempted to isolate the nightly duration, or dose, of CPAP that would restore optimal or normal daily functioning. Data from a multisite prospective cohort study of 149 newly diagnosed moderate to severe OSA participants was used to examine the nightly duration of CPAP treatment that would produce normal values in those who demonstrated excessive daytime sleepiness and functional impairment.[9] After 3 months of treatment, the greatest gains with respect to proportion of participants who obtained normal values was 4 hours for self-rated daytime sleepiness measured by the Epworth Sleepiness Scale, 6 hours for objectively measured sleepiness evaluated with the Multiple Sleep Latency Test, and 7.5 hours for functional status assessed with the Functional Outcome of Sleep Questionnaire (**Fig. 1**). Other studies have also shown that longer durations of nightly CPAP use, at least 6 hours, is associated with the restoration alertness and functioning, even in those with milder

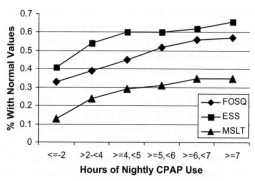

Fig. 1. Cumulative proportion of participants obtaining normal threshold values on the Epworth Sleepiness Scale, Multiple Sleep Latency Test, and Functional Outcomes of Sleep Questionnaire. (*From* Weaver TE, Maislin G, Dinges DF, et al. Relationship between hours of CPAP use and achieving normal levels of sleepiness and daily functioning. Sleep 2007;30:711–15; with permission.)

disease.[20,35,56,57] It should be noted, however, that there are a few patients who have resolution of their functional impairments with short durations of CPAP use as illustrated in **Fig. 1**. It remains unclear whether these shorter periods of use reflect total sleep time for that individual or whether it reflects individual differences in treatment response. Individual differences to sleep deprivation have been previously reported and it may be that this phenomenon also applies to response to treatment.[58,59]

WHAT ARE PREDICTORS OF ADHERENCE TO CPAP?

Among the putative factors proposed to be associated with CPAP adherence, there has been weak support for disease severity and inconsistent support for demographic characteristics, daytime sleepiness, type of device, and CPAP side effects.[16,36,60] Some patients experience claustrophobic tendencies that interfere with the ability to be optimally adherent to CPAP; however, this is true for only 15% of CPAP users.[46] Other psychological variables such as anxiety, depression, stress, anger, or social desirability do not seem to influence CPAP adherence.[61,62] However, consistent with the Sociocognitive Model of health promotion, awareness of symptoms, appreciation of the benefit of CPAP treatment following exposure, and perception that this therapy has health value has been associated with higher levels of adherence.[60,62–65] In CPAP-naïve patients, perceptions formed after commencement of therapy, in the first week of treatment, but not pretreatment, influenced CPAP use.[65,66] These perceptions were solidified with continued experience with CPAP.[66] Forty percent of social cognitive theory constructs and 33% of components of the Transtheoretical Model explained the variance in CPAP adherence at 1 month.[65] Why pretreatment cognitions do not affect CPAP adherence may be a quandary. However, application of the Sociocognitive Model presumes familiarity with the target behavior. For many patients, their first encounter with CPAP is in the middle of the night in a sleep laboratory when the mask is applied during a titration study. It is when they are faced with using the treatment on their own at home that they have the initial opportunity to acquaint themselves with the device and formulate perceptions regarding their ability to initiate treatment. This explanation is consistent with reports of a weak association between pretreatment cognitions, but stronger relationships with the commencement of therapy.[65] However, as the first week of treatment is critical in the determination of long-term adherence, an opportunity to positively affect early perceptions would be before the initiation of therapy. Indeed, there is some evidence that the initial presentation of CPAP therapy is critical to acceptance of this treatment.[67] In a study that offered a 2-week trial of CPAP, for each hour of CPAP application during this period, the likelihood of continuing CPAP at 1 year increased 1.53 times.[67] Moreover, for those who were satisfied with CPAP during this period, use was 1.49 times higher. These factors, initial trial and overall satisfaction, were predictors of continued CPAP use and those who used CPAP 2 hours or longer each night during the trial period were 18 times more likely to be using it 1 year later.[67] Additionally, in this study, participants who *perceived* a greater symptomatic improvement were three times more likely to accept CPAP long term.

Having professionals in attendance during initial introduction of CPAP treatment also appears to play a role in acceptance of this therapy. Participants in one study who underwent an attended PSG used CPAP 1 hour longer and applied it one more night than those whose CPAP exposure was unattended.[68] This study suggests that interacting with someone during the sleep study positively may influence patient perceptions. Using semistructured interviews after in-laboratory titration, another study also found that the experience during the titration night was predictive of initial problems on the first night of home use and significantly contributed to CPAP adherence.[69] The coping patterns of individuals also appear to affect persistence with this treatment. Active coping behaviors, ie, trying to aggressively solve the problem, rather than passive coping, ie, taking no planful action, were robustly associated with increased adherence.[61] Twenty percent of the variance in CPAP adherence could be accounted for by the way in which patients troubleshoot CPAP problems beyond that explained by disease severity or pretreatment level of excessive daytime sleepiness. Using confrontive and planful problem-solving approaches, rather than passive, to tackle obstacles affecting CPAP use led to more treatment success. Although untested, these data suggest that having someone available to reinforce the important benefits of this treatment, to immediately troubleshoot any mask-related problems, and to provide education and promote skill building may enhance CPAP adherence.

WHAT DO WE KNOW ABOUT PATIENT BELIEFS ABOUT OSA AND CPAP TREATMENT?

Using the Self-Efficacy Measure for Sleep Apnea (SEMSA), one study investigated OSA patients' beliefs regarding the risk imposed by OSA, whether CPAP was perceived as a benefit, and whether they could overcome common obstacles to persevere with this treatment.[70] When presented with known health and other risks associated with OSA, participants perceived that falling asleep during the day and having high blood pressure were the two risks that more than 60% of the subjects viewed as a threat associated with having OSA. However, approximately half of those asked did not acknowledge known problems associated with OSA such as problems concentrating, falling asleep while driving, or having an accident. Participants knew least about the impact of OSA on sexual desire or performance. When queried about outcomes that could be expected with CPAP treatment, responses indicated greater knowledge regarding the positive outcomes of CPAP use. More than 60% linked CPAP to feeling better, snoring less, being more active, improving the bed partner's sleep and their relationship, decreasing the chance of having a driving accident, and enhancing alertness and job performance. Consistent with their lack of appreciation of the impact of OSA on sexual functioning, only 53% felt that CPAP use would enhance sexual desire and performance. Although more than 60% indicated that they could overcome the common obstacles to CPAP use, only 58% would use CPAP if they experienced nasal stuffiness, 49% would have difficulty if it made them feel claustrophobic, and 48% would not use CPAP if it disturbed their bed partner's sleep. These data suggest that there are opportunities for educating patients regarding the health risks associated with OSA and gaps in knowledge regarding treatment benefits. It also provides some insight into obstacles that could be overcome through education, skill building, and troubleshooting to build CPAP self-efficacy.

WHAT APPROACHES HAVE BEEN USED TO IMPROVE ADHERENCE?

The pattern of adherence to CPAP treatment has not changed since it was first described 16 years ago.[37,48,49] Despite tremendous technological innovations, the problem of CPAP nonadherence has become chronic because of the failure to introduce a cost-effective intervention conceptually based and founded on variables associated with nonadherence that are applicable in clinical practice.[71] Of the few studies that have attempted interventions to improve adherence, most have used small sample sizes and all have used some form of education or reinforcement; a management strategy that is resource consuming and difficult to sustain.[72–82] For example, Hoy and colleagues[74] used an intensive approach to affect adherence that included nursing input, CPAP education at home involving the partner, hospital-based 3-night trial of CPAP, and home visits. As expected, this intervention led to significantly better CPAP use than usual care; however, application of this type of approach in the United States would be prohibitive. Improvements in technology such as auto-adjusting CPAP and flexible pressure designed to decrease the overall pressure experienced by the patient as well as humidification have not generated consistent results.[36] However, the Academy has endorsed heated humidification as a standard for CPAP therapy.[17]

Education seems like a reasonable and cost-effective method to improve adherence and has been tested in a number of studies.[73,76,80] However, with regard to merely imparting knowledge, Bandura,[83] a health promotion theorist, points out that knowledge, although a precondition for change, is insufficient to motivate change in behavior. Applying similar methodologies, the mixed results produced by these studies suggest that assumptions, rather than empirical evidence regarding the cause of nonadherence, were used as their foundation. With the insight that self-influences are needed to overcome impediments to adopting new habits and maintaining them,[83] more recent studies designed to affect self-efficacy have demonstrated improvements in CPAP adherence.[84–86] Only one of the three studies[84] (conducted only in older adults) was placebo controlled, whereas the others compared the effectiveness of the intervention with usual care.[85,86] Because change in self-efficacy following the intervention was not systematically measured in these studies, it remains unclear whether interventions developed to promote self-efficacy do in fact change perception resulting in higher levels of adherence.

HOW SHOULD CPAP TREATMENT BE EFFECTIVELY MANAGED?

The standard approach to CPAP titration remains the full-night, attended PSG performed in the laboratory, although the split-night study may be acceptable.[17] The introduction of CPAP is critical to patient acceptance. As discussed, an attended titration, where presumably there are opportunities for troubleshooting and positive reinforcement, produces a higher level of adherence than unattended studies.[68] Recently, the Centers for Disease Control and Prevention indicated that obstructive sleep apnea was a chronic disease.[87] As with any chronic disease, management should be team based using the expertise of the primary provider, sleep specialist, technologist, and nurse. As indicated in **Table 1**, education should be initiated when OSA is first suspected and ideally include the partner. Queries should be made regarding the patient's perception of the need for treatment and symptom manifestation, as lack of perception of symptoms and associated benefits of treatment may play a role in acceptance of the intervention.[60]

Patients should be given, within the constraints of reimbursement from third-party payers, the interface and device that they feel is most acceptable. There is currently considerable choice among interfaces including nasal masks, full face masks, oral-nasal interfaces, and nasal pillows. Chin straps should be considered for those who are mouth breathers or report eructation or abdominal discomfort with CPAP use. Examination of the nasal cavity for deviated septum, polyps, and other sources of obstruction should occur before the initiation of therapy, as these may contribute to feelings of claustrophobia when the mask is applied. These potential sources of obstruction can increase nasal resistance, which has been demonstrated to deter CPAP use,[88–90] and can improve treatment outcomes if resolved.[91]

As the pattern of adherence is established early and predicts long-term use,[48,49,51] and initial reporting of problems also affected the extent to which CPAP is embraced,[69] follow-up should occur early, ideally within the first week of treatment.[17] Telephone follow-up is adequate, but a postinitiation visit within the first week is best to troubleshoot mask issues, machine problems, or usage issues. CPAP use should be objectively and routinely monitored, which is a considered a treatment standard.[17] Objective data obtained from a device-based microprocessor monitor is

Table 1
Critical elements associated with CPAP adherence

Pretreatment	With Treatment Initiation
Referral source—patient, bed partner, other physician?	Heated humidification
Assessment of knowledge of OSA and perception of CPAP treatment	Phone call/follow-up first wk of treatment
Involvement of bed-partner in education and treatment initiation	Assessment of CPAP use and associated outcomes
Evaluation of patient awareness of and assessment of symptoms	Assessment of patient perception of treatment and symptom-related treatment response
How does patient handle challenges in life—active or passive problem solving	Evaluation of bed partner perception of treatment
Assessment of claustrophobic tendencies	Troubleshoot problems immediately—especially during the first week of treatment
Evaluation of nasal resistance	Evaluate for the presence of residual sleepiness and if present initiate treatment
Patient-centered mask and device selection	Retitration if presence of residual events suspected
Exposure to CPAP before initiation of therapy	

Abbreviations: CPAP, continuous positive airway pressure; OSA, obstructive sleep apnea.
(From Weaver TE. Adherence to positive airway pressure therapy. Curr Opin Pulm Med 2006;12:409–12; with permission.)

available on most devices and accessed through smartcard, modem, and Web-based applications. These data should be reviewed the first and second week and monthly thereafter. Insufficient use or changes in the pattern of use should be reviewed with the patient to ascertain the reason for these conditions. Evaluating adherence without consideration of pertinent outcomes such as daytime sleepiness or functional status, may not give an accurate picture of treatment effectiveness. As discussed above, Weaver and colleagues showed that a small proportion of patients benefit with only a few hours of CPAP treatment.[9] Therefore, the adequacy of the nightly duration of CPAP use should be viewed within the context of outcomes achieved. As indicated by the Academy, after initial CPAP set-up, long-term and yearly follow-up should be provided.[17]

When treated for OSA, most patients report less somnolence, but therapy does not always fully reverse wake impairments in individuals with severe sleepiness at presentation.[92–96] In many of these individuals, additional sources of sleepiness can be identified, such as suboptimal pressures for effective CPAP therapy; insufficient sleep time; somnolence-producing medication; or comorbidities such as pain, depression, cardiovascular disease, diabetes, or a second sleep disorder.[97] Animal models suggest that changes in the brain such as inflammatory activation, reduced extracellular dopamine levels, increased oxidative stress, gliosis, and apoptosis associated with intermittent hypoxemia, similar to OSA, may produce sleepiness.[98,99] Nonetheless, 25% of all patients who are effectively treated for OSA apnea and all other possible causes remain sleepy.[9,100–102] Thus, it is estimated that up to several million Americans once diagnosed for OSA and effectively treated will have residual sleepiness despite therapy for OSA. Several studies have demonstrated resolution of residual sleepiness with adjunctive modafinil (Provigil: Cephalon, Inc) treatment in patients where other causes of persistent sleepiness cannot be identified.[102–107]

SUMMARY

This article describes the outcomes associated with nasal CPAP treatment, significance of the issue of poor adherence in OSA, evidence regarding the optimal duration of nightly use, describes the nature and predictors of nonadherence, and presents management strategies for CPAP therapy for OSA. OSA can be effectively treated with CPAP therapy especially to improve daytime sleepiness, blood pressure, and quality of life. The major obstacle to effective treatment is adherence to this therapy. A team approach that accentuates collaboration and patient and partner involvement will be most successful in proper treatment introduction and follow-up, which should occur within the first week of treatment followed by yearly visits. Patients' use of CPAP should be routinely evaluated and problems interfering with optimal adherence adequately resolved. Modafinil treatment should be considered in those patients who experience residual sleepiness not attributable to other causes.

REFERENCES

1. Young T, Peppard PE, Gottlieb DJ. Epidemiology of obstructive sleep apnea: a population health perspective. Am J Respir Crit Care Med 2002; 165(9):1217–39.

2. Chesson AL Jr, Ferber RA, Fry JM, et al. The indications for polysomnography and related procedures. Sleep 1997;20(6):423–87.

3. National Sleep Foundation. Obstructive sleep apnea. Available at: www.sleepfoundation.org. Accessed September 2, 2009.

4. Nieto FJ, Young TB, Lind BK, et al. Association of sleep-disordered breathing, sleep apnea, and hypertension in a large community-based study. Sleep Heart Health Study. JAMA 2000;283(14): 1829–36.

5. Peppard PE, Young T, Palta M, et al. Prospective study of the association between sleep-disordered breathing and hypertension. N Engl J Med 2000; 342(19):1378–84.

6. Somers VK, White DP, Amin R, et al. Sleep apnea and cardiovascular disease: an American Heart Association/American College of Cardiology Foundation Scientific Statement from the American Heart Association Council for High Blood Pressure Research Professional Education Committee, Council on Clinical Cardiology, Stroke Council, and Council on Cardiovascular Nursing. J Am Coll Cardiol 2008;52(8):686–717.

7. Dorkova Z, Petrasova D, Molcanyiova A, et al. Effects of CPAP on cardiovascular risk profile in patients with severe obstructive sleep apnea and metabolic syndrome. Chest 2008;134:686–92.

8. Babu AR, Herdegen J, Fogelfeld L, et al. Type 2 diabetes, glycemic control, and continuous positive airway pressure in obstructive sleep apnea. Arch Intern Med 2005;165(4):447–52.

9. Weaver TE, Maislin G, Dinges DF, et al. Relationship between hours of CPAP use and achieving normal levels of sleepiness and daily functioning. Sleep 2007;30(6):711–9.

10. George CF. Sleep apnea, alertness, and motor vehicle crashes. Am J Respir Crit Care Med 2007;176(10):954–6.

11. Teran-Santos J, Jimenez-Gomez A, Cordero-Guevara J. The association between sleep apnea and the risk of traffic accidents. Cooperative Group Burgos-Santander [see comments]. N Engl J Med 1999;340(11):847–51.

12. Stradling J. Driving and obstructive sleep apnoea. Thorax 2008;63(6):481–3.

13. Hack M, Davies RJ, Mullins R, et al. Randomised prospective parallel trial of therapeutic versus subtherapeutic nasal continuous positive airway pressure on simulated steering performance in patients with obstructive sleep apnoea. Thorax 2000;55(3):224–31.

14. Westbrook PR. Sleep disorders and upper airway obstruction in adults. Otolaryngol Clin North Am 1990;23(4):727–43.

15. Sullivan CE, Grunstein RR. Continuous positive airways pressure in sleep-disordered breathing. In: Kryger MH, Roth T, Dement WC, editors. In principles and practice of sleep medicine. Philadelphia: WB Saunders; 1989. p. 559–70.

16. Gay P, Weaver T, Loube D, et al. Evaluation of positive airway pressure treatment for sleep related breathing disorders in adults. Sleep 2006;29(3):381–401.

17. Kushida CA, Littner MR, Hirshkowitz M, et al. Practice parameters for the use of continuous and bilevel positive airway pressure devices to treat adult patients with sleep-related breathing disorders. Sleep 2006;29(3):375–80.

18. Patel SR, White DP, Malhotra A, et al. Continuous positive airway pressure therapy for treating sleepiness in a diverse population with obstructive sleep apnea: results of a meta-analysis. Arch Intern Med 2003;163(5):565–71.

19. Lamphere J, Roehrs T, Wittig R, et al. Recovery of alertness after CPAP in apnea. Chest 1989;96(6): 1364–7.

20. Zimmerman ME, Arnedt JT, Stanchina M, et al. Normalization of memory performance and positive airway pressure adherence in memory-impaired patients with obstructive sleep apnea. Chest 2006;130(6):1772–8.

21. Giles TL, Lasserson TJ, Smith BH, et al. Continuous positive airways pressure for obstructive sleep apnoea in adults. Cochrane Database Syst Rev 2006;(3):CD001106.

22. Barbe F, Mayoralas LR, Duran J, et al. Treatment with continuous positive airway pressure is not effective in patients with sleep apnea but no daytime sleepiness. A randomized, controlled trial. Ann Intern Med 2001;134(11):1015–23.

23. Alajmi M, Mulgrew AT, Fox J, et al. Impact of continuous positive airway pressure therapy on blood pressure in patients with obstructive sleep apnea hypopnea: a meta-analysis of randomized controlled trials. Lung 2007;185(2):67–72.

24. Haentjens P, Van Meerhaeghe A, Moscariello A, et al. The impact of continuous positive airway pressure on blood pressure in patients with obstructive sleep apnea syndrome: evidence from

a meta-analysis of placebo-controlled randomized trials. Arch Intern Med 2007;167(8):757–64.

25. Bazzano LA, Khan Z, Reynolds K, et al. Effect of nocturnal nasal continuous positive airway pressure on blood pressure in obstructive sleep apnea. Hypertension 2007;50(2):417–23.

26. Buchner NJ, Sanner BM, Borgel J, et al. Continuous positive airway pressure treatment of mild to moderate obstructive sleep apnea reduces cardiovascular risk. Am J Respir Crit Care Med 2007; 176(12):1274–80.

27. Steiropoulos P, Papanas N, Nena E, et al. Markers of glycemic control and insulin resistance in non-diabetic patients with Obstructive Sleep Apnea Hypopnea Syndrome: does adherence to CPAP treatment improve glycemic control? Sleep Med 2009;10:887–91.

28. Cuhadaroglu C, Utkusavas A, Ozturk L, et al. Effects of nasal CPAP treatment on insulin resistance, lipid profile, and plasma leptin in sleep apnea. Lung 2009;182(2):75–81.

29. Dawson A, Abel SL, Loving RT, et al. CPAP therapy of obstructive sleep apnea in type 2 diabetics improves glycemic control during sleep. J Clin Sleep Med 2008;4(6):538–42.

30. Harsch IA, Schahin SP, Radespiel-Troger M, et al. Continuous positive airway pressure treatment rapidly improves insulin sensitivity in patients with obstructive sleep apnea syndrome. Am J Respir Crit Care Med 2004;169(2):156–62.

31. Schahin SP, Nechanitzky T, Dittel C, et al. Long-term improvement of insulin sensitivity during CPAP therapy in the obstructive sleep apnoea syndrome. Med Sci Monit 2008;14(3):CR117–21.

32. Trenell MI, Ward JA, Yee BJ, et al. Influence of constant positive airway pressure therapy on lipid storage, muscle metabolism and insulin action in obese patients with severe obstructive sleep apnoea syndrome. Diabetes Obes Metab 2007; 9(5):679–87.

33. West SD, Nicoll DJ, Wallace TM, et al. Effect of CPAP on insulin resistance and HbA1c in men with obstructive sleep apnoea and type 2 diabetes. Thorax 2007;62(11):969–74.

34. Brooks B, Cistulli PA, Borkman M, et al. Obstructive sleep apnea in obese noninsulin-dependent diabetic patients: effect of continuous positive airway pressure treatment on insulin responsiveness. J Clin Endocrinol Metab 1994;79(6):1681–5.

35. Stradling JR, Davies RJ. Is more NCPAP better? Sleep 2000;23(Suppl 4):S150–3.

36. Weaver TE, Grunstein RR. Adherence to continuous positive airway pressure therapy: the challenge to effective treatment. Proc Am Thorac Soc 2008;5(2):173–8.

37. Kribbs NB, Pack AI, Kline LR, et al. Objective measurement of patterns of nasal CPAP use by patients with obstructive sleep apnea. Am Rev Respir Dis 1993;147(4):887–95.

38. Rauscher H, Formanek D, Popp W, et al. Self-reported vs measured compliance with nasal CPAP for obstructive sleep apnea. Chest 1993;103(6): 1675–80.

39. Meurice JC, Dore P, Paquereau J, et al. Predictive factors of long-term compliance with nasal continuous positive airway pressure treatment in sleep apnea syndrome. Chest 1994;105(2):429–33.

40. Hui DS, Choy DK, Li TS, et al. Determinants of continuous positive airway pressure compliance in a group of Chinese patients with obstructive sleep apnea. Chest 2001;120(1):170–6.

41. Sanders MH, Gruendl CA, Rogers RM. Patient compliance with nasal CPAP therapy for sleep apnea. Chest 1986;90(3):330–3.

42. Sin DD, Mayers I, Man GC, et al. Long-term compliance rates to continuous positive airway pressure in obstructive sleep apnea: a population-based study. Chest 2002;121(2):430–5.

43. Massie CA, McArdle N, Hart RW, et al. Comparison between automatic and fixed positive airway pressure therapy in the home. Am J Respir Crit Care Med 2003;167(1):20–3.

44. Aloia MS, Ilniczky N, Di Dio P, et al. Neuropsychological changes and treatment compliance in older adults with sleep apnea. J Psychosom Res 2003; 54(1):71–6.

45. Bachour A, Maasilta P. Mouth breathing compromises adherence to nasal continuous positive airway pressure therapy. Chest 2004;126(4):1248–54.

46. Chasens ER, Pack AI, Maislin G, et al. Claustrophobia and adherence to CPAP treatment. West J Nurs Res 2005;27(3):307–21.

47. Lindberg E, Berne C, Elmasry A, et al. CPAP treatment of a population-based sample—what are the benefits and the treatment compliance? Sleep Med 2006;7(7):553–60.

48. Weaver TE, Kribbs NB, Pack AI, et al. Night-to-night variability in CPAP use over the first three months of treatment. Sleep 1997;20(4):278–83.

49. Budhiraja R, Parthasarathy S, Drake CL, et al. Early CPAP use identifies subsequent adherence to CPAP therapy. Sleep 2007;30(3):320–4.

50. Aloia MS, Arnedt JT, Stanchina M, et al. How early in treatment is PAP adherence established? Revisiting night-to-night variability. Behav Sleep Med 2007;5(3):229–40.

51. Rosenthal L, Gerhardstein R, Lumley A, et al. CPAP therapy in patients with mild OSA: implementation and treatment outcome. Sleep Med 2000;1(3): 215–20.

52. Krieger J. Long-term compliance with nasal continuous positive airway pressure (CPAP) in obstructive sleep apnea patients and nonapneic snorers. Sleep 1992;15(6 Suppl):S42–6.

53. McArdle N, Devereux G, Heidarnejad H, et al. Long-term use of CPAP therapy for sleep apnea/hypopnea syndrome. Am J Respir Crit Care Med 1999;159(4 Pt 1):1108–14.

54. Kribbs NB, Pack AI, Kline LR, et al. Effects of one night without nasal CPAP treatment on sleep and sleepiness in patients with obstructive sleep apnea. Am Rev Respir Dis 1993;147(5):1162–8.

55. Grunstein RR, Stewart DA, Lloyd H, et al. Acute withdrawal of nasal CPAP in obstructive sleep apnea does not cause a rise in stress hormones. Sleep 1996;19(10):774–82.

56. Engleman HM, Kingshott RN, Wraith PK, et al. Randomized placebo-controlled crossover trial of continuous positive airway pressure for mild sleep apnea/hypopnea syndrome. Am J Respir Crit Care Med 1999;159(2):461–7.

57. Barnes M, Houston D, Worsnop CJ, et al. A randomized controlled trial of continuous positive airway pressure in mild obstructive sleep apnea. Am J Respir Crit Care Med 2002;165(6):773–80.

58. Van Dongen HP, Maislin G, Mullington JM, et al. The cumulative cost of additional wakefulness: dose-response effects on neurobehavioral functions and sleep physiology from chronic sleep restriction and total sleep deprivation. Sleep 2003;26(2):117–26.

59. Van Dongen HP, Maislin G, Dinges DF. Dealing with inter-individual differences in the temporal dynamics of fatigue and performance: importance and techniques. Aviat Space Environ Med 2004; 75(3 Suppl):A147–54.

60. Engleman HM, Wild MR. Improving CPAP use by patients with the sleep apnoea/hypopnoea syndrome (SAHS). Sleep Med Rev 2003;7(1):81–99.

61. Stepnowsky CJ Jr, Bardwell WA, Moore PJ, et al. Psychologic correlates of compliance with continuous positive airway pressure. Sleep 2002;25(7): 758–62.

62. Wells RD, Freedland KE, Carney RM, et al. Adherence, reports of benefits, and depression among patients treated with continuous positive airway pressure. Psychosom Med 2007;69(5):449–54.

63. Weaver TE. Predicting adherence to continuous positive airway pressure—the role of patient perception. J Clin Sleep Med 2005;1(4):354–6.

64. Wild MR, Engleman HM, Douglas NJ, et al. Can psychological factors help us to determine adherence to CPAP? A prospective study. Eur Respir J 2004;24(3):461–5.

65. Stepnowsky C, Marler M, Ancoli-Israel S. Determinants of nasal CPAP compliance. Sleep Med 2002;3:239–47.

66. Aloia MS, Arnedt JT, Stepnowsky C, et al. Predicting treatment adherence in obstructive sleep apnea using principles of behavior change. J Clin Sleep Med 2005;1(4):346–53.

67. Popescu G, Latham M, Allgar V, et al. Continuous positive airway pressure for sleep apnoea/hypopnoea syndrome: usefulness of a 2 week trial to identify factors associated with long term use. Thorax 2001;56(9):727–33.

68. Means MK, Edinger JD, Husain AM. CPAP compliance in sleep apnea patients with and without laboratory CPAP titration. Sleep Breath 2004;8(1):7–14.

69. Lewis KE, Seale L, Bartle IE, et al. Early predictors of CPAP use for the treatment of obstructive sleep apnea. Sleep 2004;27(1):134–8.

70. Weaver TE, Maislin G, Dinges DF, et al. Self-efficacy in sleep apnea: instrument development and patient perceptions of obstructive sleep apnea risk, treatment benefit, and volition to use continuous positive airway pressure. Sleep 2003;26(6):727–32.

71. Haniffa M, Lasserson TJ, Smith I. Interventions to improve compliance with continuous positive airway pressure for obstructive sleep apnoea. Cochrane Database Syst Rev 2004;(4):CD003531.

72. Fletcher EC, Luckett RA. The effect of positive reinforcement on hourly compliance in nasal continuous positive airway pressure users with obstructive sleep apnea. Am Rev Respir Dis 1991;143:936–41.

73. Chervin RD, Theut S, Bassetti C, et al. Compliance with nasal CPAP can be improved by simple interventions. Sleep 1997;20(4):284–9.

74. Hoy CJ, Vennelle M, Kingshott RN, et al. Can intensive support improve continuous positive airway pressure use in patients with the sleep apnea/hypopnea syndrome? Am J Respir Crit Care Med 1999;159(4 Pt 1):1096–100.

75. Meurice JC, Marc I, Series F. Efficacy of auto-CPAP in the treatment of obstructive sleep apnea/hypopnea syndrome. Am J Respir Crit Care Med 1996;153(2):794–8.

76. Hui DS, Chan JK, Choy DK, et al. Effects of augmented continuous positive airway pressure education and support on compliance and outcome in a Chinese population. Chest 2000; 117(5):1410–6.

77. DeMolles DA, Sparrow D, Gottlieb DJ, et al. A pilot trial of a telecommunications system in sleep apnea management. Med Care 2004;42(8):764–9.

78. Stepnowsky CJ, Palau JJ, Marler MR, et al. Pilot randomized trial of the effect of wireless telemonitoring on compliance and treatment efficacy in obstructive sleep apnea. J Med Internet Res 2007;9(2):e14.

79. Smith CE, Dauz ER, Clements F, et al. Telehealth services to improve nonadherence: a placebo-controlled study. Telemed J E Health 2007;12: 289–96.

80. Wiese HJ, Boethel C, Phillips B, et al. CPAP compliance: video education may help! Sleep Med 2005; 6:171–4.

81. Meurice JC, Ingrand P, Portier F, et al. A multicentre trial of education strategies at CPAP induction in the treatment of severe sleep apnoea-hypopnoea syndrome. Sleep Med 2007;8:37–42.

82. Golay A, Girard A, Grandin S, et al. A new educational program for patients suffering from sleep apnea syndrome. Patient Educ Couns 2006;60:220–7.

83. Bandura A. Health promotion by social cognitive means. Health Educ Behav 2004;31(2):143–64.

84. Aloia MS, Dio LD, Ilniczky N, et al. Improving compliance with nasal CPAP and vigilance in older adults with OSAHS. Sleep Breath 2001;5(1):13–22.

85. Aloia MS, Smith K, Arnedt JT, et al. Brief behavioral therapies reduce early positive airway pressure discontinuation rates in sleep apnea syndrome: preliminary findings. Behav Sleep Med 2007;5(2):89–104.

86. Richards D, Bartlett DJ, Wong K, et al. Increased adherence to CPAP with a group cognitive behavioral treatment intervention: a randomized trial. Sleep 2007;30(5):635–40.

87. Centers for Disease Control and Prevention Division of Adult and Community Health (DACH). Sleep and sleep disorders: a Public Health Challenge. Available at: http://www.cdc.gov/sleep/index.htm. Accessed July 25, 2009.

88. Li HY, Engleman H, Hsu CY, et al. Acoustic reflection for nasal airway measurement in patients with obstructive sleep apnea-hypopnea syndrome. Sleep 2005;28(12):1554–9.

89. Morris LG, Burschtin O, Lebowitz RA, et al. Nasal obstruction and sleep-disordered breathing: a study using acoustic rhinometry. Am J Rhinol 2005;19(1):33–9.

90. Sugiura T, Noda A, Nakata S, et al. Influence of nasal resistance on initial acceptance of continuous positive airway pressure in treatment for obstructive sleep apnea syndrome. Respiration 2007;74(1):56–60.

91. Nakata S, Noda A, Yagi H, et al. Nasal resistance for determinant factor of nasal surgery in CPAP failure patients with obstructive sleep apnea syndrome. Rhinology 2005;43(4):296–9.

92. Engleman HM, Martin SE, Deary IJ, et al. Effect of continuous positive airway pressure treatment on daytime function in sleep apnoea/hypopnoea syndrome. Lancet 1994;343(8897):572–5.

93. Meurice JC, Paquereau J, Neau JP, et al. Long-term evolution of daytime somnolence in patients with sleep apnea/hypopnea syndrome treated by continuous positive airway pressure. Sleep 1997;20(12):1162–6.

94. Tiihonen M, Partinen M. Polysomnography and maintenance of wakefulness test as predictors of CPAP effectiveness in obstructive sleep apnea. Electroencephalogr Clin Neurophysiol 1998;107(6):383–6.

95. Kingshott RN, Vennelle M, Hoy CJ, et al. Predictors of improvements in daytime function outcomes with CPAP therapy. Am J Respir Crit Care Med 2000;161(3 Pt 1):866–71.

96. Ellen RL, Marshall SC, Palayew M, et al. Systematic review of motor vehicle crash risk in persons with sleep apnea. J Clin Sleep Med 2006;2(2):193–200.

97. Santamaria J, Iranzo A, Ma Montserrat J, et al. Persistent sleepiness in CPAP treated obstructive sleep apnea patients: evaluation and treatment. Sleep Med Rev 2007;11(3):195–207.

98. Zhu Y, Fenik P, Zhan G, et al. Selective loss of catecholaminergic wake active neurons in a murine sleep apnea model. J Neurosci 2007;27(37):10060–71.

99. Gozal D, Daniel JM, Dohanich GP. Behavioral and anatomical correlates of chronic episodic hypoxia during sleep in the rat. J Neurosci 2001;21(7):2442–50.

100. Guilleminault C, Philip P. Tiredness and somnolence despite initial treatment of obstructive sleep apnea syndrome (what to do when an OSAS patient stays hypersomnolent despite treatment). Sleep 1996;19(9 Suppl):S117–22.

101. Morisson F, Decary A, Petit D, et al. Daytime sleepiness and EEG spectral analysis in apneic patients before and after treatment with continuous positive airway pressure. Chest 2001;119(1):45–52.

102. Pack AI, Black JE, Schwartz JR, et al. Modafinil as adjunct therapy for daytime sleepiness in obstructive sleep apnea. Am J Respir Crit Care Med 2001;164(9):1675–81.

103. Schwartz J, Schwartz E, Veit C, et al. Modafinil as an adjunctive therapy for excessive daytime somnolence in obstructive sleep apnea. Sleep 2000;23(Suppl 2):A85.

104. Dinges DF, Weaver TE. Effects of modafinil on sustained attention performance and quality of life in OSA patients with residual sleepiness while being treated with nCPAP. Sleep Med 2003;4(5):393–402.

105. Black JE, Hirshkowitz M. Modafinil for treatment of residual excessive sleepiness in nasal continuous positive airway pressure-treated obstructive sleep apnea/hypopnea syndrome. Sleep 2005;28(4):464–71.

106. Schwartz JR, Hirshkowitz M, Erman MK, et al. Modafinil as adjunct therapy for daytime sleepiness in obstructive sleep apnea: a 12-week, open-label study. Chest 2003;124(6):2192–9.

107. Bittencourt LR, Lucchesi LM, Rueda AD, et al. Placebo and modafinil effect on sleepiness in obstructive sleep apnea. Prog Neuropsychopharmacol Biol Psychiatry 2008;32(2):552–9.

Principles of Oral Appliance Therapy for the Management of Snoring and Sleep Disordered Breathing

Fernanda R. Almeida, DDS, MSc, PhD[a],*,
Alan A. Lowe, DMD, DipOrtho, PhD[b]

KEYWORDS
- Oral appliance (OA) • Mandibular repositioning appliance
- Tongue retaining device • Treatment • Snoring
- Sleep apnea

OVERVIEW OF ORAL APPLIANCES

Oral appliance (OA) therapy for snoring, obstructive sleep apnea (OSA), or both is simple, reversible, quiet, and cost-effective and may be indicated in patients who are unable to tolerate nasal continuous positive airway pressure (nCPAP) or are poor surgical risks. OAs are effective in varying degrees and seem to work because of an increase in airway space, the provision of a stable anterior position of the mandible, advancement of the tongue or soft palate, and possibly a change in genioglossus muscle activity. The appliances should be used during sleep for life and must be comfortable for the patient. Finally, OAs can only be used in cooperative patients who are motivated to wear the appliance during sleep on a regular basis.

OA therapy falls into two main categories: those that hold the tongue forward and those that reposition the mandible (and the attached tongue) forward during sleep. Before treating either snoring or OSA with any OA, a complete assessment by a physician experienced in the field or by a sleep disorder specialist is important. After concluded that treatment with an OA is indicated, the physician provides the dentist/orthodontist/oral and maxillofacial surgeon who has skill and experience in OA therapy with a written referral or prescription and a copy of the diagnostic report. Because of the obvious life-threatening implications of several sleep disorders, OA therapy must commence only after a complete medical assessment.

The American Academy of Sleep Medicine (AASM) reviewed the available literature in 2006 and recommended that OAs may be used as first line therapy in adult patients with primary snoring, mild and moderate OSA and in patients with severe OSA who are intolerant of or refuse treatment with nasal nCPAP.[1,2] For some patients, combination therapy with other treatments such as weight loss, surgery and nCPAP may be indicated, and this must be coordinated by the attending sleep physician.

OAs for the treatment of snoring and OSA have proven to be effective in reducing the apnea-hypopnea index (AHI) and increasing minimum oxygen saturation,[3–8] further improving sleep architecture[6] and reducing arousals.[6,8,9] Subjectively and objectively, OAs decrease sleepiness to the same degree as nCPAP,[7,10–13] decrease objectively measured snoring in most patients,[6,7] and improve

[a] Department of Oral Biological and Medical Sciences, The University of British Columbia, 2199 Wesbrook Mall, Vancouver, BC V6T 1Z3, Canada
[b] Division of Orthodontics, Department of Oral Health Sciences, The University of British Columbia, 2199 Wesbrook Mall, Vancouver, BC V6T 1Z3, Canada
* Corresponding author.
E-mail address: falmeida@interchange.ubc.ca (F.R. Almeida).

Oral Maxillofacial Surg Clin N Am 21 (2009) 413–420
doi:10.1016/j.coms.2009.07.002
1042-3699/09/$ – see front matter Crown Copyright © 2009 Published by Elsevier Inc. All rights reserved.

quality of life and neuropsychological function.[14,15] Moreover, OAs have been shown to improve cardiovascular health[9,12,16,17] and driving performance.[13,18]

Since the first publication of the AASM position papers,[19,20] two significant advances in this field have occurred: adjustable appliances that allow titration of the mandibular position over time, and the use of materials and designs that significantly improve intraoral retention. Dentists realized early that determining the correct jaw position was the most difficult step when using OA therapy successfully. Patients had considerable variations in the initial comfortable range of the anteroposterior movement of the mandible, and differences in the speed and amount of forward jaw position that could be tolerated. Single jaw position or nonadjustable appliances often must be remade if the initial jaw position proves to be inadequate. Gradual titration forward of the mandible without needing a new appliance to be made each time became the objective, and adjustable appliances were invented and marketed.

A subgroup of patients, particularly those experiencing sleep bruxism,[21] often experience a considerable jaw discomfort in the morning after wearing a rigid hard acrylic single jaw position OA. A need to develop an OA that could allow for lateral jaw movement and some degree of vertical jaw opening was identified. Concurrently, major advances in dental materials significantly improved the flexibility and strength of thermosensitive acrylic resin materials. Appliances made of temperature-sensitive material that patients could heat in hot water before insertion that would cool and harden somewhat intraorally were found to have considerably more retention than traditionally designed cold-cure acrylic appliances. The combination of adjustability, lateral and vertical jaw movement, increased retention, and better-defined titration protocols have significantly improved the effectiveness of OA since they were first systematically reviewed.

Each OA has a primary effect on either the tongue or the tongue and mandible together. Several appliances move the mandible anteriorly, such as Somnomed (Denton, TX), Klearway (Tonawanda, NY), elastomeric (Tonawanda, NY) single jaw position appliances, Herbst (Tonawanda, NY), TAP III (Dallas, TX), and PM Positioner (Tonawanda, NY), (Fig. 1). The tongue is affected by all appliances, either through direct forward movement of the muscle itself or changes secondary to an altered mandibular rest position. The tongue retaining device is the most commonly used OA that has a direct affect on tongue posture.

Despite the in-depth research in the field of pediatric sleep medicine, little is known about the efficacy and side effects of OAs for children who have no craniofacial abnormalities.[22,23] Orthodontic treatment for children who have OSA and craniofacial anomalies has shown to be effective not only for dentition but also in decreasing

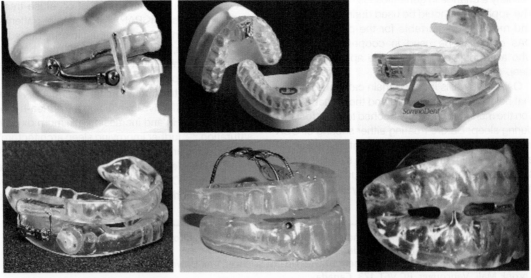

Fig. 1. Lateral views of six oral appliances used for the treatment of snoring or obstructive sleep apnea. Herbst (Tonawanda, NY), Tap III (Dallas, TX), Somnomed (Denton, TX), PM Positioner (Tonawanda, NY), Klearway (Tonawanda, NY), and Elastomeric (Tonawanda, NY), single jaw position appliances. (Courtesy of Somnomed Inc, Great Lakes Orthodontics, Dr M. Marklund, Dr J. Parker, Airway Managment Inc.)

respiratory disturbances in children.[24,25] This article focuses on the use of OAs in the adult population only.

This article provides a detailed clinical protocol and titration sequence for OAs, because this clinical procedure is often not well understood by practitioners new to the field. Prediction of treatment success is addressed, OA treatment is compared with surgery and nCPAP, OA compliance is described, and the possible adverse effects associated with this type of therapy are discussed.

CLINICAL PROTOCOL FOR ORAL APPLIANCE THERAPY

The following therapy sequence is suggested for the management of OAs in patients who are being treated for snoring or OSA.

1. Medical assessment is completed by the attending physician or sleep specialist. Before referral to a dentist, the physician should check that the patient has sufficient teeth (at least eight in each of the upper and lower jaws) and that they have no limitations in forward jaw movement (>5 mm) or jaw opening (>25 mm). Totally edentulous patients may not be ideally suited for treatment with mandibular repositioners because they may not have enough intraoral retention to keep the appliance in the mouth during sleep. Patients who have edentulous maxillary arches and adequate teeth in the lower arch may experience favorable response to mandibular repositioners. Full upper and lower dentures may preclude the use of a mandibular repositioner, but some of these patients may experience a good treatment response with a tongue retaining device. Partial dentures that replace four or fewer teeth do not preclude OA use. Evidence of a severe history of temporomandibular joint (TMJ) pathology or chronic joint pain may preclude the use of an OA in some patients. In patients who have mild to moderate TMJ disorders, OAs may be used if the patient is instructed to systematically perform TMJ support therapy exercises.[26] Severe occlusal wear (>20% of the clinical crown) may indicate severe bruxism and complicate OA therapy if the grinding persists. Prediction of OA success is described further in this article.

2. An overnight polysomnogram with a detailed evaluation of the diagnostic criteria for OSA must be completed by the physician or sleep specialist before treatment with an OA is initiated. Written referral or prescription and a diagnostic report are sent to a dentist or dental specialist.

3. An oral examination is completed and includes medical and dental histories. Careful assessments are completed of soft tissue structures, periodontal status, TMJ, occlusion, intraoral habits and the teeth and restorations. Initial dental radiographs, such as panoramic or full mouth survey; cephalometric radiograph (optional); and diagnostic plaster models are important records of the dentist's initial assessment.

4. Appliance determination is made, which includes consideration of mandibular repositioner versus tongue retainer and whether a boil-and-bite type or a custom-made appliance is required.

5. After fabrication, the dentist should fit the appliance and adjust for patient comfort. The patient must then be instructed and trained as how to manage the appliance.

6. If an adjustable OA is used, the dentist should follow up with the patient during the period of titration. Details of a titration protocol are outlined later. Possible need for modification, redesign, or remake of an OA is based on subjective resolution of symptoms, patient compliance, and a follow-up sleep study.

7. The patient should be referred back to attending physician for assessment or repeat overnight sleep study. The objective assessment of OA efficacy is recommended because evidence shows that OAs may have a placebo effect on OSA symptoms.[5,7] During the polysomnogram, further OA titration may be useful.

8. If the OA has been shown to be effective and the patient is comfortable, the attending dentist should schedule recall appointments every 6 months for the first 2 years. At each appointment, the status of the occlusion should be checked. The dentist should also monitor subjective effectiveness, fit, comfort, TMJ, and dental status.

9. Regular follow-up appointments must be scheduled at least once a year to monitor OA wear, efficacy, and possible adverse effects. OAs are known to last approximately 2 to 3 years. If the appliance is showing extensive wear, such as cracks, discoloration, or lost of retention, a new appliance is recommended. The dentist may have to advance the appliance further if symptoms recur. If maximum mandibular advancement is reached and symptoms are still present, the patient must be referred to the sleep specialist for further evaluation. A careful evaluation of the occlusion is necessary and patients must be advised of the probability of occlusal changes.

TITRATION PROTOCOLS

Once the patient wears the appliance every night and is comfortable for one month, he or she should be instructed to start advancing the appliance. As an example for discussion, we describe the titration of a specific screw mechanism, but the concept is similar for most of the adjustable appliances. When using the Hyrax screw, present in Klearway, PM Positioner, Somnomed appliance, titration is accomplished by turning the screw two times per week until the next appointment. Each turn or activation in the direction of the arrow moves the lower jaw gradually forward in 0.25-mm increments, which has a direct effect on the three-dimensional size of the airway. The patient inserts the tip of the key into the hole on the side of the expansion screw at the base of the arrow and turns or pushes the key toward the direction of the arrow imprinted in the metal expansion screw, which shows the correct movement to advance the lower jaw Once the key is completely turned from one side to the other it is removed, and a new hole appears for the next turn. If the key is removed before a new hole appears after the completed turn, the patient may be unable to fully place the key in the new hole. The key is always removed after turning. Turning the key opposite to the direction of the arrow closes the expansion screw and retracts the mandible. If significant jaw or joint discomfort occurs, advise the patient to stop turning the screw until their next visit.

Some patients stop snoring and feel more rested shortly after the appliance is inserted, and no further advancement of the mandible is required. Others may require 2 or 3 months of slow and gradual forward repositioning before a significant treatment effect is noted. When the patient or bed partner reports a cessation of snoring and a resolution of symptoms, further advancement of the mandible may not be required and the appliance is considered titrated. The expansion screw should be tied off with stainless steel ligature wire or filled in with cold cure acrylic to prevent any further movement of the screw. The patient should be referred back to his or her physician or sleep specialist for assessment at this time.

The efficacy of titration and timing of a repeat polysomnogram for OA titration are factors in OA therapy that still require further understanding. Krishnan and colleagues[27] showed that although 55% of patients achieve successful self-titration at home, another 32% can reach success with further polysomnography-guided titration. Almeida and colleagues[28] also showed that titration at night can improve results of the usual clinical advancement of the OA by up to 35%. The protocol is simple to implement in the sleep laboratory, with the technologist asking the patient to advance the appliance in 1-mm increments if the patient continued to snore, showed increased respiratory effort, or had ongoing respiratory events. Patients should not be awakened more than three times to achieve a sufficient sleep time during the titration polysomnogram despite being awakened to make the advancements.

COMPLIANCE AND ADVERSE EFFECTS

The compliance and side effects of OA treatment might differ depending on the type of the appliance, disease severity, and perhaps patient management. Compliance is often measured subjectively, except in one study in which a compliance monitor indicated that the OA was worn for a mean of 6.8 hours per night.[11] A greater percentage of noncompliant patients is seen in the first 6 months, with approximately 40% of noncompliant patients identified during this period.[29]

The most common reasons to stop using the appliance are discomfort/cumbersome (46%) and no or little effect (36%). Compliance rates vary widely among studies, with a minimum of 4% to a maximum of 82% of compliance after 1 year of treatment.[30,31] In a study involving 630 patients, Marklund and colleagues[32] described compliance among 75% of the patients after 12 months of treatment. After 2 to 5 years of follow-up, studies have shown compliance rates of 48% up to 90%.[12,33–36] One study reported an adherence drop from 82% to 62% from year 1 to 4.[14] Studies with nCPAP have shown that subjective compliance is often higher than objective assessment; therefore, until a compliance monitor is available for OA therapy follow-up, caution should be taken when evaluating OA compliance.

The main reasons for discontinuing treatment are reported to be insufficient reduction of snoring and the presence of side effects.[29] Most side effects caused by OAs are usually described as mild and transient, and most frequently include dry mouth, excessive salivation, mouth or teeth discomfort, muscle tenderness, and jaw stiffness. Significant and persistent TMJ problems are rare.[2] One study used MRI to evaluate the TMJ of seven patients over a mean period of 11 months, concluding that OA in the titrated position seem to be innocuous to the TMJ in patients who have OSA.[10]

Long-term side effects were more recently described in evaluating OA side effects over a period of more than 5 years. Using a titratable appliance (Klearway) Almeida and colleagues[37,38] showed that OAs used for a mean period of 7.3 years have a significant impact on occlusal and dental structures (eg, a 2.8 mm decrease in overbite and a 2.6 mm decrease in overjet). Changes observed in craniofacial structures were mainly related to significant tooth movements. Marklund[39] observed that the frequent use of a monoblock OA with full occlusal coverage for 5 years resulted in median reductions in overjet and overbite of 0.6 mm in patients who had snoring and OSA. Infrequent users had smaller bite changes. Overjet decreased during the first and second halves of the treatment period, and overbite changes diminished with time.

Although some occlusal changes might be undesirable in certain patients, the effective treatment of a life-threatening disease such as OSA seems to supersede the maintenance of a baseline occlusion. All therapies exhibit side effects, and OAs are no exception.

PREDICTION OF TREATMENT SUCCESS

The OA treatment protocol varies from nCPAP, especially as it applies to titration. Because patients may not be able to initially tolerate the mandibular advancement required to open the airway during sleep, OAs cannot be easily tried for a single night to predict treatment success and patient compliance. OAs require up to 6 months of gradual titration to be fully adjusted. Previous research has evaluated whether overnight titration of mandibular advancement during polysomnography could be used to initiate OA therapy similar to the titration of nCPAP.[40–43] The first study of overnight titration used an OA that was removed from the patient's mouth and adjusted manually.[40] Other titration studies have used a temporary appliance that can be adjusted either by waking the patient[43] or without waking the patient.[41,42] The temporary appliance was advanced either manually after removal of the temporary appliance,[43] using a hydraulic system,[41] or through remote control of a motorized system.[42] Results of these studies were mixed in terms of predicting the amount of advancement needed for successful OA therapy. Furthermore, overnight titration of an OA remains an experimental approach, and the technology for remote controlled advancement is not widely available.

One study used a prefabricated boil-and-bite appliance as a screening tool for OA therapy.[44] This randomized, controlled, crossover study found that a prefabricated appliance had a compliance failure rate of 31%, whereas a custom-made appliance showed only a 6% rate of compliance failure. The prefabricated appliance showed an exceptionally high total failure rate of 69%, whereas the failure rate of the custom-made appliance was 40%. This study concluded that custom-made appliances cannot be recommended as a therapeutic option nor can they be used as a screening tool to identify good candidates for OA therapy.

Clinical, physiologic, and polysomnographic variables have been identified as predictors of success in many research studies. Clinically, younger patients[45,46] who have a lower AHI,[5,32,46,47] a smaller neck circumference,[5] a lower body mass index (BMI),[46,48] and positional OSA[32,49] have shown higher success rates with OA therapy. Correlations exist between OA success and the amount of mandibular advancement, with greater advancement exhibiting the highest decrease in AHI and oxygen desaturation index.[10,50] Women have shown a higher success rate than men.[32]

OA success has also been linked to some cephalometric characteristics, such as a shorter palate, a larger retropalatal airway space, a decreased distance between the hyoid and mandibular plane, a narrow anteroposterior position of mandible (SNB) angle, and a higher anteroposterior position of maxilla (SNA) angle.[5,51–53] Using MRI during the Müller maneuver, together with mandibular advancement, one study found a correlation between an improvement in upper airway patency and treatment success.[54] More recently, physiologic assessments of nasal resistance and pulmonary function were shown to have some predictive value.[55–57]

Even with all the variables described, most studies have been underpowered, and no prospective study could define patient characteristics to accurately predict treatment outcome. Therefore, further studies are needed before treatment success or treatment failure can be predicted before the 6 months of OA titration is initiated.

COMPARATIVE EFFECTIVENESS OF ORAL APPLIANCES, NASAL CONTINUOUS POSITIVE AIRWAY PRESSURE, AND SURGERY

Only one study compares OAs with upper airway surgery (uvulopalatopharyngoplasty [UPPP]), with subsequent reports on the same patient pool.[14,30,58,59] This study[59] was a randomized parallel study that treated 45 patients with an OA and 43 with UPPP. At the 1-year follow-up, OA showed a higher success rate in controlling the AHI than UPPP (78% vs 51%). Both treatments were equally effective in reducing sleepiness, although the surgical group showed greater contentment. Of the participating patients, 32 treated with OA and 40 treated with UPPP completed the 4-year follow-up.[14] Both groups showed an increase in BMI, and no significant correlation was seen between changes in BMI and AHI from baseline to the 4-year follow-up within the OA and UPPP groups.

According to the criteria for OSA (apnea index $\geq$ 5 or AHI $\geq$ 10), 63% of patients in the dental appliance group attained normalization after 4 years, a proportion that was significantly higher than the 33% among patients in the UPPP group. Three patients in the UPPP group showed a tendency to fibrotic narrowing, but without symptoms. Pronounced complaints of nasopharyngeal regurgitation of fluid and difficulty with swallowing after UPPP were reported by 8% and 10%, respectively. In the OA group, 22 patients did not notice any changes in tooth contacts and 4 noted minor changes. One patient was not able to occlude his teeth in the same way as before treatment and reported TMJ discomfort. OA side effects were described as minor and infrequent.[58] In conclusion, the group treated with an OA showed a significantly higher success and normalization rate than the group treated with UPPP.

Seven randomized controlled trials recently showed the efficacy of OA against nCPAP.[4,8,16,47,60–62] When only AHI is evaluated, nCPAP is consistently superior to OA: in six of seven studies, nCPAP normalized the AHI, whereas OA failed to do so in a third or more of the patients.

Even though the AHI was better controlled with nCPAP, no difference was seen in objective sleepiness or neurobehavioral outcomes between the therapies. One explanation could be the hours of use and acceptance of treatment. Treatment preference is complex and depends on variables such as patient age and lifestyle. In five studies, OAs were preferred over nCPAP treatment, whereas in one no preference was seen[62] and in one the patients preferred nCPAP over an OA.[16] In conclusion, nCPAP is more effective than OA in reducing AHI, but with respect to improvements in symptoms, compliance with and acceptance of OAs are similar to those for nCPAP.

REFERENCES

1. Kushida CA, Morgenthaler TI, Littner MR, et al. Practice parameters for the treatment of snoring and obstructive sleep apnea with oral appliances: an update for 2005. Sleep 2006;29(2):240–3.
2. Ferguson KA, Cartwright R, Rogers R, et al. Oral appliances for snoring and obstructive sleep apnea: a review. Sleep 2006;29(2):244–62.
3. Cartwright RD, Samelson CF. The effects of a nonsurgical treatment for obstructive sleep apnea. The tongue-retaining device. JAMA 1982;248(6):705–9.
4. Ferguson KA, Ono T, Lowe AA, et al. A short-term controlled trial of an adjustable oral appliance for the treatment of mild to moderate obstructive sleep apnoea. Thorax 1997;52(4):362–8.
5. Mehta A, Qian J, Petocz P, et al. A randomized, controlled study of a mandibular advancement splint for obstructive sleep apnea. Am J Respir Crit Care Med 2001;163(6):1457–61.
6. Pitsis AJ, Darendeliler MA, Gotsopoulos H, et al. Effect of vertical dimension on efficacy of oral appliance therapy in obstructive sleep apnea. Am J Respir Crit Care Med 2002;166(6):860–4.
7. Gotsopoulos H, Chen C, Qian J, et al. Oral appliance therapy improves symptoms in obstructive sleep apnea: a randomized, controlled trial. Am J Respir Crit Care Med 2002;166(5):743–8.
8. Tan YK, L'Estrange PR, Luo YM, et al. Mandibular advancement splints and continuous positive airway pressure in patients with obstructive sleep apnoea: a randomized cross-over trial. Eur J Orthod 2002; 24(3):239–49.
9. Gotsopoulos H, Kelly JJ, Cistulli PA. Oral appliance therapy reduces blood pressure in obstructive sleep apnea: a randomized, controlled trial. Sleep 2004; 27(5):934–41.
10. de Almeida FR, Bittencourt LR, de Almeida CI, et al. Effects of mandibular posture on obstructive sleep apnea severity and the temporomandibular joint in patients fitted with an oral appliance. Sleep 2002; 25(5):507–13.
11. Lowe AA, Sjoholm TT, Ryan CF, et al. Treatment, airway and compliance effects of a titratable oral appliance. Sleep 2000;23(Suppl 4):S172–8.
12. Yoshida K. Effects of a mandibular advancement device for the treatment of sleep apnea syndrome and snoring on respiratory function and sleep quality. Cranio 2000;18(2):98–105.
13. Hoffstein V. Review of oral appliances for treatment of sleep-disordered breathing. Sleep Breath 2007; 11(1):1–22.
14. Walker-Engstrom ML, Tegelberg A, Wilhelmsson B, et al. 4-year follow-up of treatment with dental appliance or uvulopalatopharyngoplasty in patients with obstructive sleep apnea: a randomized study. Chest 2002;121(3):739–46.
15. Naismith S, Winter V, Gotsopoulos H, et al. Neurobehavioral functioning in obstructive sleep apnea: differential effects of sleep quality, hypoxemia and subjective sleepiness. J Clin Exp Neuropsychol 2004;26(1):43–54.
16. Barnes M, McEvoy RD, Banks S, et al. Efficacy of positive airway pressure and oral appliance in mild to moderate obstructive sleep apnea. Am J Respir Crit Care Med 2004;170(6):656–64.

17. Otsuka R, Ribeiro de Almeida F, Lowe AA, et al. The effect of oral appliance therapy on blood pressure in patients with obstructive sleep apnea. Sleep Breath 2006;10(1):29–36.

18. Hoekema A, Stegenga B, Bakker M, et al. Simulated driving in obstructive sleep apnoea-hypopnoea; effects of oral appliances and continuous positive airway pressure. Sleep Breath 2007; 11(3):129–38.

19. Schmidt-Nowara W, Lowe A, Wiegand L, et al. Oral appliances for the treatment of snoring and obstructive sleep apnea: a review. Sleep 1995;18(6): 501–10.

20. Practice parameters for the treatment of snoring and obstructive sleep apnea with oral appliances. American Sleep Disorders Association. Sleep 1995;18(6): 511–3.

21. Sjoholm TT, Lowe AA, Miyamoto K, et al. Sleep bruxism in patients with sleep-disordered breathing. Arch Oral Biol 2000;45(10):889–96.

22. Nelson S, Kulnis R. Snoring and sleep disturbance among children from an orthodontic setting. Sleep Breath 2001;5(2):63–70.

23. Carvalho FR, Lentini-Oliveira D, Machado MA, et al. Oral appliances and functional orthopaedic appliances for obstructive sleep apnoea in children. Cochrane Database Syst Rev 2007;(2): CD005520.

24. Pirelli P, Saponara M, Guilleminault C. Rapid maxillary expansion in children with obstructive sleep apnea syndrome. Sleep 2004;27(4):761–6.

25. Cozza P, Polimeni A, Ballanti F. A modified monobloc for the treatment of obstructive sleep apnoea in paediatric patients. Eur J Orthod 2004;26(5):523–30.

26. Cunali PA, Almeida FR, Santos CD, et al. Influence in the quality of life and efficacy of support therapy for TMD as an adjunct therapy for OA treatment. Sleep Breath 2008;12(4):408.

27. Krishnan V, Collop NA, Scherr SC. An evaluation of a titration strategy for prescription of oral appliances for obstructive sleep apnea. Chest 2008;133(5): 1135–41.

28. Almeida FR, Parker J, Hodges J, et al. Effect of a titration polysomnogram on treatment success with a mandibular repositioning appliance. J Clin Sleep Med 2009;5(3):198–204.

29. de Almeida FR, Lowe AA, Tsuiki S, et al. Long-term compliance and side effects of oral appliances used for the treatment of snoring and obstructive sleep apnea syndrome. J Clin Sleep Med 2005; 1(2):143–52.

30. Walker-Engstrom ML, Wilhelmsson B, Tegelberg A, et al. Quality of life assessment of treatment with dental appliance or UPPP in patients with mild to moderate obstructive sleep apnoea. A prospective randomized 1-year follow-up study. J Sleep Res 2000;9(3):303–8.

31. Nakazawa Y, Sakamoto T, Yasutake R, et al. Treatment of sleep apnea with prosthetic mandibular advancement (PMA). Sleep 1992;15(6):499–504.

32. Marklund M, Stenlund H, Franklin KA. Mandibular advancement devices in 630 men and women with obstructive sleep apnea and snoring: tolerability and predictors of treatment success. Chest 2004; 125(4):1270–8.

33. Clark GT, Sohn JW, Hong CN. Treating obstructive sleep apnea and snoring: assessment of an anterior mandibular positioning device. J Am Dent Assoc 2000;131(6):765–71.

34. Marklund M, Sahlin C, Stenlund H, et al. Mandibular advancement device in patients with obstructive sleep apnea: long-term effects on apnea and sleep. Chest 2001;120(1):162–9.

35. Menn SJ, Loube DI, Morgan TD, et al. The mandibular repositioning device: role in the treatment of obstructive sleep apnea. Sleep 1996;19(10): 794–800.

36. Pantin CC, Hillman DR, Tennant M. Dental side effects of an oral device to treat snoring and obstructive sleep apnea. Sleep 1999;22(2):237–40.

37. Almeida FR, Lowe AA, Otsuka R, et al. Long-term sequellae of oral appliance therapy in obstructive sleep apnea patients: part 2. Study-model analysis. Am J Orthod Dentofacial Orthop 2006;129(2): 205–13.

38. Almeida FR, Lowe AA, Sung JO, et al. Long-term sequellae of oral appliance therapy in obstructive sleep apnea patients: part 1. Cephalometric analysis. Am J Orthod Dentofacial Orthop 2006;129(2): 195–204.

39. Marklund M. Predictors of long-term orthodontic side effects from mandibular advancement devices in patients with snoring and obstructive sleep apnea. Am J Orthod Dentofacial Orthop 2006; 129(2):214–21.

40. Raphaelson MA, Alpher EJ, Bakker KW, et al. Oral appliance therapy for obstructive sleep apnea syndrome: progressive mandibular advancement during polysomnography. Cranio 1998;16(1): 44–50.

41. Petelle B, Vincent G, Gagnadoux F, et al. One-night mandibular advancement titration for obstructive sleep apnea syndrome: a pilot study. Am J Respir Crit Care Med 2002;165(8):1150–3.

42. Tsai WH, Vazquez JC, Oshima T, et al. Remotely controlled mandibular positioner predicts efficacy of oral appliances in sleep apnea. Am J Respir Crit Care Med 2004;170(4):366–70.

43. Kuna ST, Giarraputo PC, Stanton DC, et al. Evaluation of an oral mandibular advancement titration appliance. Oral Surg Oral Med Oral Pathol Oral Radiol Endod 2006;101(5):593–603.

44. Vanderveken OM, Devolder A, Marklund M, et al. Comparison of a custom-made and a thermoplastic

oral appliance for the treatment of mild sleep apnea. Am J Respir Crit Care Med 2008;178(2):197–202.

45. Liu Y, Park YC, Lowe AA, et al. Supine cephalometric analyses of an adjustable oral appliance used in the treatment of obstructive sleep apnea. Sleep Breath 2000;4(2):59–66.

46. Liu Y, Lowe AA, Fleetham JA, et al. Cephalometric and physiologic predictors of the efficacy of an adjustable oral appliance for treating obstructive sleep apnea. Am J Orthod Dentofacial Orthop 2001;120(6):639–47.

47. Clark GT, Blumenfeld I, Yoffe N, et al. A crossover study comparing the efficacy of continuous positive airway pressure with anterior mandibular positioning devices on patients with obstructive sleep apnea. Chest 1996;109(6):1477–83.

48. Cartwright RD. Predicting response to the tongue retaining device for sleep apnea syndrome. Arch Otolaryngol 1985;111(6):385–8.

49. Yoshida K. Influence of sleep posture on response to oral appliance therapy for sleep apnea syndrome. Sleep 2001;24(5):538–44.

50. Kato J, Isono S, Tanaka A, et al. Dose-dependent effects of mandibular advancement on pharyngeal mechanics and nocturnal oxygenation in patients with sleep-disordered breathing. Chest 2000; 117(4):1065–72.

51. Eveloff SE, Rosenberg CL, Carlisle CC, et al. Efficacy of a Herbst mandibular advancement device in obstructive sleep apnea. Am J Respir Crit Care Med 1994;149(4 Pt 1):905–9.

52. Mayer G, Meier-Ewert K. Cephalometric predictors for orthopaedic mandibular advancement in obstructive sleep apnoea. Eur J Orthod 1995; 17(1):35–43.

53. Otsuka R, Almeida FR, Lowe AA, et al. A comparison of responders and nonresponders to oral appliance therapy for the treatment of obstructive sleep apnea. Am J Orthod Dentofacial Orthop 2006;129(2):222–9.

54. Sanner BM, Heise M, Knoben B, et al. MRI of the pharynx and treatment efficacy of a mandibular advancement device in obstructive sleep apnoea syndrome. Eur Respir J 2002;20(1):143–50.

55. Ng AT, Qian J, Cistulli PA. Oropharyngeal collapse predicts treatment response with oral appliance therapy in obstructive sleep apnea. Sleep 2006; 29(5):666–71.

56. Zeng B, Ng AT, Darendeliler MA, et al. Use of flow-volume curves to predict oral appliance treatment outcome in obstructive sleep apnea. Am J Respir Crit Care Med 2007;175(7):726–30.

57. Zeng B, Ng AT, Qian J, et al. Influence of nasal resistance on oral appliance treatment outcome in obstructive sleep apnea. Sleep 2008;31(4):543–7.

58. Tegelberg A, Wilhelmsson B, Walker-Engstrom ML, et al. Effects and adverse events of a dental appliance for treatment of obstructive sleep apnoea. Swed Dent J 1999;23(4):117–26.

59. Wilhelmsson B, Tegelberg A, Walker-Engstrom ML, et al. A prospective randomized study of a dental appliance compared with uvulopalatopharyngoplasty in the treatment of obstructive sleep apnoea. Acta Otolaryngol 1999;119(4):503–9.

60. Ferguson KA, Ono T, Lowe AA, et al. A randomized crossover study of an oral appliance vs nasal-continuous positive airway pressure in the treatment of mild-moderate obstructive sleep apnea. Chest 1996;109(5):1269–75.

61. Randerath WJ, Heise M, Hinz R, et al. An individually adjustable oral appliance vs continuous positive airway pressure in mild-to-moderate obstructive sleep apnea syndrome. Chest 2002;122(2):569–75.

62. Engleman HM, McDonald JP, Graham D, et al. Randomized crossover trial of two treatments for sleep apnea/hypopnea syndrome: continuous positive airway pressure and mandibular repositioning splint. Am J Respir Crit Care Med 2002;166(6): 855–9.

Sleep Apnea Surgery: Putting It All Together

Kasey K. Li, MD, DDS, FACS

KEYWORDS
- Maxillomandibular advancement
- Sleep surgery • Uvulopalatopharyngoplasty
- Sleep apnea • Sleep apnea surgery

Since the first description of uvulopalatopharyngo-plasty (UPPP) in 1972,[1] the surgical management of obstructive sleep apnea syndrome (OSA) has become increasingly popular. This popularity is caused by several reasons. The psychomotor sequelae of OSA, such as excessive daytime sleepiness, daytime fatigue, and poor sleep quality caused by sleep fragmentation, have major dele-terious impact on patients' well being,[2,3] which behooves them to seek treatment. The risk of hypertension,[4,5] heart attack,[6] and stroke[7] also prompts patients to seek treatment. Further, despite the potential success of nasal continuous positive airway pressure (CPAP),[8,9] patients' compliance represents a clear problem,[10,11] thus causing patients to seek treatment alternatives, namely surgery.

Despite the wide acceptance of sleep apnea surgery within surgical specialties of oral and maxil-lofacial surgery and otolaryngology, many sleep physicians remain skeptical on the efficacy of sleep apnea surgery. Publications have been critical of surgery regarding its outcome.[12,13] However, the conclusions of these articles have been flawed and unrealistic in the realm of patients' care. For example, Elshaug and colleagues[13] proposed that "all future surgical audits report objective cure rates with success based on apnea-hypopnea index (AHI) outcomes of less than or equal to five or less than or equal to 10." However, nasal CPAP, which is the first line and considered to be the gold standard treatment, establishes acceptable compliance of 4 hours per night and 70% of the nights. This compliance rate represents only approximately 50% of ideal use.[14] Therefore, nasal CPAP incompletely eliminates sleep-related breathing disorder and clearly does not satisfy the criteria recommended by Elshaug and colleagues[13] for surgery. One needs to realize that OSA is similar to chronic illness, such as dia-betes or hypertension, as the total elimination of these diseases is impossible. Therefore, the goal of any treatment modality is to improve or control the symptoms and the risk of OSA by reducing the severity. Sleep apnea surgery clearly satisfies that goal. The commonly accepted criteria for surgical success, which achieves a 50% reduction of respiratory disturbance index and below 20 events per hour, is certainly reasonable.

In examining the outcomes of sleep apnea surgery, one of the glaring problems is the predict-ability of surgery. The success of UPPP has been quoted to be approximately 40%.[15] However, the success rate of any type of sleep apnea surgery is influenced by factors, such as the severity of the sleep apnea, body mass index, airway anatomy, and ethnicity. Even in evaluating the outcomes of maxillomandibular advancement (MMA), which is considered the most successful surgery for OSA, one will find that the success rate ranges from 57% to the mid 90% range.[16–18] To improve the predictability of surgical success, many preoperative assessments have been advo-cated to evaluate the airway, including cephalo-metric analysis, fiberoptic nasopharyngoscopy with or without Mueller's maneuver, CT, MRI, fluoroscopy, and sleep endoscopy. Additionally, phased surgical protocol has been used by many surgeons with the intent to minimize the amount of surgery performed in any one phase, thus mini-mizing the risk of unnecessary surgery. Such phased protocol begins with the less invasive

Multidisciplinary Treatment Team, Stanford Sleep Disorders Clinic and Research Center, 1900 University Avenue, Suite # 105, Stanford, CA 94303, USA
E-mail address: drli@sleepapneasurgery.com

Oral Maxillofacial Surg Clin N Am 21 (2009) 421–423
doi:10.1016/j.coms.2009.08.003

surgery, such as UPPP, nasal surgery, genioglossus advancement, hyoid advancement, and radiofrequency, and MMA is only offered as the last resort.[16,19] On the other hand, some surgeons advocate MMA as the sole treatment modality and only offer UPPP when necessary, after MMA.[20]

When the author first started treating patients who have OSA, they had followed the phased protocol because it sounded conservative and patients prefer the less invasive procedures to control their problem. After a few years, the author realized that the adherence of any protocol in sleep apnea surgery is inadequate in the management of many patients; in fact, it often results in unnecessary procedures. One should realize that the phase protocol was established over 20 years ago. A tremendous amount of knowledge has been acquired since that time. We now have sufficient data and experience to know that patients who have severe OSA, minimal pharyngeal soft-tissue redundancy, absence of tonsillar tissues, and significant maxillomandibular deficiency are simply going to have a low response rate to less invasive surgical procedures. In these patients, the only procedure that will achieve a sufficient success rate is MMA. However, patients who have favorable factors, such as significant tonsillar hypertrophy, low body mass index, and mild to moderate OSA can be offered phased protocol because the chance of success with the initial phase is acceptable. These patients should not be convinced to undergo MMA simply because it is the only procedure that the surgeon performs. All surgeons treating patients who have OSA must realize that the management of OSA crosses specialty lines and no single specialty can adequately take care of patients alone. Oral and maxillofacial surgeons and otolaryngologists must establish collaborative efforts in properly counseling patients regarding their surgical options, providing legitimate success rate of the procedures, and discussing surgical risks. This collaboration is the only way that sleep apnea surgery will be recognized as a legitimate treatment option by the established field of sleep medicine and provides our patients with quality and predictable options.

REFERENCES

1. Fijita S, Conway W, Zorick F, et al. Surgical correction of anatomic abnormalities of obstructive sleep apnea syndrome: uvulopalatopharyngoplasty. Otolaryngol Head Neck Surg 1981;89:923–34.

2. Gottlieb DJ, Whitney CW, Bonekat WH, et al. Relation of sleepiness to respiratory disturbance index: the Sleep Heart Health Study. Am J Respir Crit Care Med 1999;159:502–7.

3. Young T, Paltz M, Dempsey J, et al. The occurrence of sleep-disordered breathing among middle-aged adults. N Engl J Med 1993;328:1230–5.

4. Nieto FJ, Young TB, Lind BK, et al. Association of sleep-disordered breathing, sleep apnea, and hypertension in a large community-based study. Sleep Heart Health Study. JAMA 2000;283:1829–36.

5. Peppard PE, Young T, Palta M, et al. Prospective study of the association between sleep-disordered breathing and hypertension. N Engl J Med 2000;342:1378–84.

6. Peker Y, Kraiczi H, Hedner J, et al. An independent association between obstructive sleep apnoea and coronary artery disease. Eur Respir J 1999;14:179–84.

7. Shamsuzzaman AS, Somers VK. Fibrinogen, stroke, and obstructive sleep apnea: an evolving paradigm of cardiovascular risk [editorial]. Am J Respir Crit Care Med 2000;162:2018–20.

8. Jenkinson C, Davies RJ, Mullins R, et al. Comparison of therapeutic and subtherapeutic nasal continuous positive airway pressure for obstructive sleep apnoea: a randomized prospective parallel trial. Lancet 1999;353:2100–5.

9. Hack M, Davies RJ, Mullins R, et al. Randomised prospective parallel trial of therapeutic versus subtherapeutic nasal continuous positive airway pressure on simulated steering performance in patients with obstructive sleep apnoea. Thorax 2000;55:224–31.

10. Kribbs NB, Redline S, Smith PL, et al. Objective monitoring of nasal CPAP usage in OSAS patients. J Sleep Res 1991;20:270–1.

11. ElReeves-Hoche MK, Meck R, Zwillich CW. Nasal CPAP: an objective evaluation of patient compliance. Am J Respir Crit Care Med 1994;149:149–54.

12. Elshaug AG, Moss JR, Southcott AM, et al. An analysis of the evidence-practice continuum: is surgery for obstructive sleep apnoea contraindicated? J Eval Clin Pract 2007;13:3–9.

13. Elshaug AG, Moss JR, Southcott AM, et al. Redefining success in airway surgery for obstructive sleep apnea: a meta analysis and synthesis of the evidence. Sleep 2007;30:461–7.

14. Grote L, Hedner J, Grunstein R, et al. Therapy with nCPAP: incomplete elimination of sleep related breathing disorder. Eur Respir J 2000;16:921–7.

15. Sher AE, Schechtman KB, Piccirillo JF. The efficacy of surgical modifications of the upper airway in adults with obstructive sleep apnea syndrome. Sleep 1996;19:156–77.

16. Hendler BH, Costello BJ, Silverstein K, et al. A protocol for uvulopalatopharyngoplasty, mortised genioplasty, and maxillomandibular advancement in patients with obstructive sleep apnea: an analysis of 40 cases. J Oral Maxillofac Surg 2001;59:892–7.

17. Li KK, Riley RW, Powell NB, et al. Obstructive sleep apnea surgery: patients' perspective and polysomnographic results. Otolaryngol Head Neck Surg 2000;123:572–5.

18. Li KK, Powell NB, Riley RW, et al. Overview of phase II surgery for obstructive sleep apnea syndrome. Ear Nose Throat J 1999;78:851–7.

19. Riley RW, Powell NB, Guilleminault C. Maxillofacial surgery and obstructive sleep apnea: a review of 80 patients. Otolaryngol Head Neck Surg 1989; 101(3):353–61.

20. Hochban W, Conradt R, Brandenburg U, et al. Surgical maxillofacial treatment of obstructive sleep apnea. Plast Reconstr Surg 1997;99:619–26.

Anesthetic and Postoperative Management of the Obstructive Sleep Apnea Patient

Samuel A. Mickelson, MD, FACS, ABSM[a,b,]*

KEYWORDS

- Complications • OSAS surgery
- Obstructive sleep apnea • Anesthesia
- Post op management
- Avoid complications in sleep apnea surgery

Clinically significant obstructive sleep apnea hypopnea syndrome (OSAHS) occurs in 4% of men and 2% of women[1] and is caused by a decrease in upper airway size and patency during sleep. During sleep, a patient may develop a complete obstruction of the airway (apnea), partial obstruction of the airway leading to a desaturation or arousal from sleep (hypopnea), or partial obstruction of the airway leading to an arousal but no significant desaturation (respiratory effort–related arousal). Although the number of these respiratory events per hour (respiratory disturbance index [RDI]) of sleep is currently used as the determinant of sleep apnea severity (**Table 1**), this disease leads to morbidity and mortality because of the physiologic consequences of the respiratory events rather than as a direct result of the respiratory events. These physiologic changes include reductions in oxygen saturation, increases in sympathetic output and tone, hypercarbia, and arousals from sleep. Arousals lead to cessation of the respiratory event, only to be followed by repetitive airflow obstructions and arousals. The arousals cause sleep fragmentation and secondary daytime symptoms, including nonrestorative sleep, excessive daytime somnolence, and problems with concentration and memory. Arousals also led to a rise in sympathetic tone, with secondary increases in blood pressure, pulse, and cardiac output. The reduction of oxygen saturation can directly lead to cardiac arrhythmias, myocardial infarction, and stroke.

Safe perioperative management of patients with obstructive sleep apnea requires special attention to preoperative, intraoperative, and postoperative care. Sleep apnea is a common condition and may be present even if a planned surgical procedure is not being performed for this indication. These patients are more likely to have comorbidities, including hypertension, insulin resistance, diabetes, coronary artery disease, gastroesophageal and laryngopharyngeal reflux disease, and obesity.

These patients typically have anatomic features (retrognathia, micrognathia, macroglossia, tonsil and uvula hypertrophy, nasal obstruction, abnormal epiglottis position, anterior positioning of the larynx, or elongation of the airway) that may lead to difficulty with intraoperative ventilation and intubation. Apnea severity may worsen after

[a] Advanced Ear Nose & Throat Associates PC, Atlanta, GA 30342, USA
[b] The Atlanta Snoring and Sleep Disorders Institute, 960 Johnson Ferry Road, Suite 200, Atlanta, GA 30342, USA
* Corresponding author. The Atlanta Snoring and Sleep Disorders Institute, 960 Johnson Ferry Road, Suite 200, Atlanta, GA 30342.
E-mail address: sammickelson@earthlink.net

Oral Maxillofacial Surg Clin N Am 21 (2009) 425–434
doi:10.1016/j.coms.2009.08.002
1042-3699/09/$ – see front matter © 2009 Elsevier Inc. All rights reserved.

Table 1
Sleep apnea severity

	RDI	LSAT
Mild	5–14	86%–90%
Moderate	15–29	70%–85%
Severe	>30	<70%

The American Academy of Sleep Medicine currently recommends use of the RDI in determination of sleep apnea severity. RDI is defined as the total number of apneas, hypopneas, and respiratory effort–related arousals during the study divided by the number of hours of recorded sleep. In contrast, the Apnea Hypopnea Index is defined as the total number of apneas and hypopneas during the study divided by the number of hours of recorded sleep.

Abbreviation: LSAT, lowest oxygen saturation.

surgery due to a combination of these anatomic features along with airway edema caused by a difficult intubation or due to drug effects leading to a reduction of the arousal response. Anesthetic agents, narcotic analgesics, and sedative hypnotics reduce the brain's arousal response and may lengthen respiratory events and worsen hypoxemia and hypercarbia during sleep. These factors may predispose to postoperative airway obstruction and, ultimately, myocardial infarction, stroke, cardiac arrhythmia, and sudden death.

There is growing evidence that sleep apnea is a risk factor for anesthesia-related morbidity and mortality. These risks are present when undergoing any surgical procedure, including upper airway surgery. The care of these patients requires vigilance before, during, and after surgery to minimize risks associated with their underlying diseases. This article reviews potential complications from surgery along with avoidance strategies.

PREOPERATIVE CONSIDERATIONS
Selection of a Surgical Facility

When operating on patients with obstructive sleep apnea, surgeons must select a facility with personnel and equipment adequate for an elective and controlled management of patient airway before and after the procedure. Unfortunately, there is insufficient literature to offer guidance regarding which patients can be safely managed on an outpatient as opposed to an inpatient basis or how long patients need to be monitored postoperatively.[2] Most publications suggest, however, that patients with more severe sleep apnea are at greater risk for perioperative complications. The concern is not the number of respiratory

events per hour but rather the degree of oxygen desaturation, because patients with severe desaturation have minimal respiratory reserve and are already on the steep-sloped portion of the oxygen desaturation curve.

Surgery may be performed in an office, outpatient surgery center, or hospital operating room. After surgery, patients may be monitored in a recovery unit for a short or extended time, transferred to a 23- to 48-hour observation unit, transferred to the hospital by ambulance, or admitted to a regular hospital room, a room with telemetry, or an intensive care unit (ICU). The choice of surgical setting and postoperative setting is best determined preoperatively[2] and should be made after consideration of associated comorbidities, severity of apnea, sites of airway narrowing, type of anesthesia and surgery, anticipated length of surgery, and need for postoperative narcotic agents. Consultants to the American Society of Anesthesiologists[2] were surveyed using a nonvalidated scoring system about opinions regarding "outpatient surgery" in patients with OSAHS. Their opinions were that patients with mild sleep apnea undergoing uvulopalatopharyngoplasty (UPPP) or nasal surgery were not at increased risk for complications, whereas patients with moderate sleep apnea undergoing UPPP were at increased risk of complications.[2] The goal of postoperative monitoring is to document severity of the sleep apnea and oxygen desaturation in patients while they are sleeping without supplemental oxygen, so they can be treated it, if needed, thereby preventing complications.

Hospital policies and protocols and the quality of the hospital nursing care can also have an impact on the level and type of postoperative monitoring. For example, some facilities can perform continuous pulse oximetry in an extended recovery unit whereas others require an ICU for the same level of care. It is the author's opinion that nonairway surgery in most patients with mild or moderate sleep apnea may be done safely only as outpatient, whereas those with severe sleep apnea or undergoing pharyngeal surgery require some observation, preferably with time observed while asleep, before discharge. When performing surgery for reasons other than sleep apnea, the same issues need to be considered.

Choice of Anesthesia Technique (Local, General, or Monitored Anesthesia Care)

There is insufficient literature to evaluate the effects of different anesthetic techniques on surgical complications in patients with OSAHS. Because airway reconstructive surgery for sleep apnea causes blood to enter the airway, it is typically felt to be safest to perform these surgeries while patients are intubated, to control and protect the airway. When patients with sleep apnea are undergoing nonairway surgery, then local anesthesia, or monitored anesthesia care may be preferred. Sedation must be performed carefully, as sleep apnea patients are more sensitive to sedatives, causing more muscle relaxation and prolongation of respiratory events. When using conscious sedation, continuous pulse oximetry, cardiac monitoring, and CO_2 monitoring should be used. General anesthesia with a secure airway is preferred if patients require moderate or deep sedation.

Use of Preoperative Continuous Positive Airway Pressure

Before surgery, patients are often sleep deprived due to anxiety about the upcoming surgery. In those with poor positive airway pressure (positive airway pressure [PAP], continuous PAP [CPAP], bilevel positive airway pressure [BiPAP], or auto-PAP) compliance, sleep deprivation persists.[3,4] Once surgery is completed, however, patients are likely to have a rebound of delta and rapid eye movement sleep and may be predisposed to more severe sleep apnea.[5] It is likely that measures that can improve sleep quality prior to surgery may reduce the rebound of deep sleep postoperatively. Although most patients undergoing sleep apnea reconstructive surgery are doing so because they are poorly compliant with PAP, even modest use of PAP prior to surgery may be beneficial. If PAP is available, patients should be asked to use their machine for several weeks prior to and after surgery and to bring their machine into the hospital for perioperative use.

Use of Narcotics and Sedative Agents

Routine use of sedative hypnotics, anxiolytic agent, and narcotics should be avoided prior to surgery in patients with obstructive sleep apnea syndrome (OSAHS) as these agents may lead to sudden death, even in a preoperative holding area.[6] Narcotics suppress respiratory drive, blunt the arousals response, and may lead to life-threatening hypoxemia. Benzodiazepine agonists reduce upper airway dilator muscle tone and worsen sleep-disordered breathing.[7] Flurazepam increases the apnea index[8] whereas triazolam reduces oxygen saturation and the arousal response and increases the duration of respiratory events.[9] If sleep apnea patients require one of these drugs immediately prior to surgery, they

should be monitored with continuous pulse oximetry and may require supplemental oxygen.

Reflux/Aspiration Precautions

Obesity is common in patients with OSAHS and is associated with increased intra-abdominal fat, higher intra-abdominal pressure, and a higher incidence of hiatal hernia and gastroesophageal reflux.[10,11] Obese patients have a larger volume of gastric fluid and a lower gastric pH and are at increased risk of aspiration during induction of anesthesia[12] or on extubation. To reduce these risks, obese patients should receive an H_2 blocker, proton pump inhibitor, or esophageal motility stimulant prior to surgery,[13] and the stomach should be suctioned out during or on completion of surgery.

Preoperative Medical Clearance

Consultation with a primary physician, cardiologist, anesthesiologist, or other appropriate specialists should be considered in patients with complicated comorbid conditions or multiple comorbidities. Medical issues that may warrant medical clearance include hypertension requiring multiple medications, poorly controlled diabetes, coronary artery disease, cerebrovascular disease, or underlying pulmonary disease. The purpose of the preoperative clearance is to optimize control of the comorbidities prior to surgery and, hopefully, reduce the risk of surgical complications. Patients with OSAHS have a higher prevalence of hypertension due to an increased sympathetic output during respiratory events.[14,15] Blood pressure should be checked prior to surgery and, if significantly elevated, these patients should be referred for treatment prior to surgery.

Communication with the Anesthesia Team

As the head of the surgical team, it is the surgeon's responsibility to communicate with the anesthesia team about any potential difficulties that may arise during surgery. The anesthesiologist should be told about the severity of the sleep apnea and any upper airway abnormalities, such as macroglossia, retrognathia, or micrognathia, that could pose a challenge to ventilate, intubate, or secure an airway. In these patients, a surgeon may request to have difficult airway tools or a tracheostomy set in the operating room.

INTRAOPERATIVE CONSIDERATIONS
Patient Ventilation

An antireflux agent and antisialogogue should be administered preoperatively to reduce the risk of aspiration and excess saliva production.[13] After induction of anesthesia, patients require positive pressure breathing by mask, head, and neck extension; jaw protrusion; and insertion of a properly sized oral airway or long nasal airway that can extend beyond the tongue base. A two-person ventilation approach may be needed, one for jaw positioning and mask seal and the other for squeezing the bag.[16] A variety of methods are available to maintain ventilation of a difficult airway (**Box 1**). The simplest approach is to insert a long oral airway or nasopharyngeal airway that extends below the tongue base. A laryngeal mask airway (LMA) is another excellent way to stabilize the airway and allow ventilation.[17,18] The LMA is inserted blindly, keeping the base of tongue and epiglottis from collapsing posteriorly. A 3- to 5-minute period of ventilation is used to increase oxyhemoglobin saturation prior to intubation.

Intubation Techniques

Sleep apnea patients can be a challenge to intubate due to the combination of mandibular or maxillary deficiency, a long floppy airway, excessive oropharyngeal and hypopharyngeal soft tissue, and a relatively anterior larynx. If easily ventilated, then short-acting paralyzing agents, such as succinylcholine, may be used prior to intubation. If the larynx cannot be visualized, alternative methods (**Box 2**) may be required.

New techniques have mostly replaced the older approaches of awake oral or nasal intubation and a planned awake transnasal fiberoptic intubation performed with patients in a sitting or semisitting position. The newer options allow patients to be asleep before intubation but should be reserved for patients who are likely to have no problems with ventilation. New techniques include use of a light wand (lighted stilet) inserted into the endotracheal tube, with transcutaneous guidance into the trachea, in a darkened room. Other options include ventilation through an LMA, then intubation

Box 2
Available methods for difficult intubation
Awake intubation
Light wand
Fiberoptic intubation
Video laryngoscopes
Intubation through LMA
Retrograde intubation
Blind nasal intubation

through the LMA. The newest development is the video laryngoscope (currently marketed as the GlideScope, Burnaby British Columbia, Canada), which uses a small video camera on the end of a curved laryngoscope Mac blade, allowing an anesthesiologist to visualize the larynx on a screen and then guide the endotracheal tube through the vocal cords. The advantage of the technique is the ability to view the larynx "around the corner" in patients who have micrognathia or retrognathia and an anteriorly positioned larynx. One disadvantage is the large size of the blade, making it difficulty to insert in patients with trismus.

A planned tracheostomy should be considered in those with severe sleep apnea, failure of CPAP, life-threatening cardiac arrhythmias, severe oxygen desaturation,[19] or failed intubation at a prior surgery or if significant postoperative airway edema is expected. An emergency tracheostomy or cricothyrotomy may be needed if patients cannot be ventilated or intubated.

Extubation

Another critical time for airway complications is extubation. Before extubation, anesthesiologists should verify full reversal of neuromuscular blockade; patients should have purposeful movement, recovery of neuromuscular activity, sustainable head lift for at least 5 seconds, and an adequate voluntary tidal volume. Ventilation is typically easier for patients in the semiupright or lateral position. Patients should be extubated with appropriate personnel and equipment present so as to be able to replace the tube if necessary. It is generally accepted that patients should be extubated awake[2,20] because if patients are still "deep," the airway may obstruct. When performing upper airway surgery, however, if extubated light or awake, patients may cough or buck on the tube and cause bleeding into the airway. The decision to extubate light or deep, therefore, is made by the surgeon and anesthesiologist. If

Box 1
Available methods for difficult ventilation
Oral airway
Long nasopharyngeal airways
LMA
Esophageal-tracheal combitube
Rigid ventilating bronchoscope
Intratracheal jet stylet
Transtracheal jet ventilation

patients were easy to ventilate with induction, and surgery did not cause significant airway edema, then there should be no difficulty ventilating after extubation.

It is unclear whether or not use of local anesthetic agents effect safety. Use of a long-acting local anesthetic during surgery may reduce the need for narcotic analgesics but may worsen apnea due to their effect on airway mechanoreceptors that contribute to the arousal stimulus and apnea termination.[21] Narcotic agents should be minimized during surgery, as their effect may persist postoperatively leading to postoperative complications.

Surgeon Availability

A surgeon and anesthesiologist should both be in the operating room at time of induction, intubation, and extubation for all sleep apnea patients.

POSTOPERATIVE CONSIDERATIONS
Postoperative Monitoring

Several studies have shown that when all healed, reconstructive surgery improves apnea severity, but sleep apnea is typically unchanged or worse for the first two nights.[22,23] It is believed that the first 24 hours after surgery is the most critical time for complications, although postoperative deaths have occurred later, most commonly due to the accumulated effects of sleep deprivation, narcotic agents, and rapid eye movement rebound.[24,25] Unfortunately, the literature is insufficient to offer guidance about how long monitoring is needed or if there is any preferred type of monitoring: standard hospital room, telemetry unit, ICUs, or intermediate ICUs.[2]

The reason for postoperative monitoring is early detection or prevention of complications. Continuous pulse oximetry with an audible alarm is the easiest and most reliable method for early detection of postoperative hypoventilation. Intermittent oximetry monitoring has minimal benefit for this patient population because patients usually are awakened by putting on the oximetry probe and, once awake, would not be having apnea. Continuous pulse oximetry should be used for all OSAHS patients after nonairway surgery or upper airway reconstructive surgery. Although there is no consensus as to whether or not electrocardiographic monitoring is beneficial for those with sleep apnea, it should be considered in patients with significant cardiac disease or arrhythmias.

Most older publications have recommended monitoring oxygen saturation and cardiac arrhythmias in the ICU[22,26] whereas others have advocated ICU monitoring due to the high reported incidence of serious airway complications (13%–25%) after UPPP.[27,28] Older studies suggest that ICU monitoring may decrease the risk of complications after OSAS surgery.[27,29] More recent publications, however, note a much lower risk of airway complications (1.4%), likely due to more aggressive perioperative treatment of tissue edema and avoidance of excessive sedation.[30–32] Except for the sickest of sleep apnea patients and those undergoing maxillomandibular advancement, the author believes that ICU monitoring is rarely required for soft tissue surgeries.

Many surgeons, anesthesiologists, and hospitals have standard protocols governing preoperative and postoperative standard orders before and after surgery.[33] Institution and anesthesia protocols should be reviewed to verify that routine recovery room, surgical ward, or extended recovery unit orders are appropriate for the sleep apnea patient (**Boxes 3** and **4**). In general, monitoring of vital signs for sleep apnea patients should be more frequent than for patients without OSAHS. Nursing checks should specifically monitor for respiratory rate, depth of breathing, and presence of snoring and to verify that there is no apnea, hypopnea, or labored breathing.

Patient Positioning

The apnea hypopnea index and hypoxemia tend to improve when these patients sleep in the lateral or

---

Box 3
Standard preoperative orders for sleep apnea surgery

1. Famotidine (or other H_2 receptor antagonist) __ mg by mouth 30 to 60 minutes before surgery

2. Metaclopramide __ mg by mouth 30 to 60 minutes before surgery

3. Glycopyrrolate (or other anticholinergic agent) __ mg intramuscularly (IM) 30 to 60 minutes before surgery

4. Cephazolin (or other appropriate antibiotic) __ mg intravenously (IV) piggy-back (PB) 30 to 60 minutes before surgery

5. Dexamethasone sodium phosphate __ mg IV 30 to 60 minutes before surgery

6. Oxymetazoline nasal spray, __ sprays each nostril, given 10 to 20 minutes preoperatively if patients are to undergo nasal surgery or nasal intubation

7. No narcotic or sedative agents given before surgery

Box 4
Standard postoperative orders after sleep apnea surgery

1. Recovery room orders: no IV or IM narcotics 30 minutes before transfer to room

2. Try to wean oxygen to room air; maintain O_2 saturation above 90%

3. Vitals: per recovery room, then routine

4. Check patient breathing effort and record results at least every 2 hours

5. Continuous pulse oximetry

6. Elevate head of bed 30° to 45°

7. Ice collar to neck as needed

8. Sequential compression stockings to be on while in bed

9. Clear liquid diet; advance as tolerated; encourage oral intake; monitor oral intake

10. IV dextrose 5% in lactated Ringer's injection at __ mL per hour

11. Cefazolin (or other appropriate antibiotic) __ mg IVPB every 8 hours

12. Chlorhexidine, 0.5-oz swish and spit 3 times a day (if patient had palate or base of tongue surgery)

13. Patients are to wear their own CPAP/BiPAP machine, whenever sleeping, beginning in recovery room. If patient underwent nasal surgery, use a CPAP/BiPAP full face mask. Do not use CPAP/BiPAP if patient underwent maxillary or mandibular advancement.

14. For pain:

    1. Chloroseptic spray to oral cavity as needed, keep at bedside

    2. Mild: hydrocodone/acetaminophen elixer 2.5/166 mg/5 mL; contains 2–5 mg of hydrocodone and 166 mg of acetaminophen, as an elixir in each 5 mL of solution. __ mL by mouth every 6 hours as needed

    3. Moderate: oxycodone/acetaminophen elixer 5/325 mg/5 mL: contains 5 mg of oxycodone and 325 mg of acetaminophen, as an elixir in each 5 mL of solution. __ mL by mouth every 6 hours as needed

    4. Severe: nalbuphine hydrochloride __ mg IM or slow IV every 3 to 6 hours as needed.

15. Dexamethasone sodium phosphate __ mg IVPB at __ PM today and __ AM tomorrow

16. Oxymetazoline nasal spray: __ sprays to each nostril every 8 hours

17. For blood pressure elevation: systolic greater than 160 or ciastolic greater than 90 give

    1. Hydralazine HCl __ mg IV (if heart rate [HR] <80); may repeat every 15 minutes × 4 doses total

    2. Labetalol HCl __ mg IV (if HR >80); may repeat every 15 minutes × 4 doses total

18. Cough, deep breathing and incentive spirometry every 2 hours while awake

19. Call physician for:

    1. Active bleeding from nose or mouth

    2. Any evidence of respiratory distress

    3. Oxygen saturation below 90% or inability to wean off supplemental oxygen

    4. Temperature above 101° (oral)

    5. Systolic BP greater than 160, diastolic greater than 90, not controlled with prescribed medication

---

prone positions or with head of bed elevated. Sleep apnea tends to be worse when supine, due to posterior collapse of the base of tongue. After surgery, elevation of the head of the bed reduces soft tissue edema and turbinate swelling and reduces nasal airway resistance. Because there are no valves in the veins of the head and neck, lying flat increases venous pressure and worsens tissue edema. Although the literature is insufficient to provide definitive guidance in the postoperative period, most physicians agree that after airway surgery, the head of bed should be elevated and the supine position should be avoided.[2] Sleep positioning maneuvers should be recommended in the hospital and after discharge to home.

Postoperative Analgesia

Opiates drugs (morphine, meperedine, hydromorphone, fentanyl, and so forth) lead to a dose-dependent reduction of respiratory drive, respiratory rate, and tidal volume, causing hypoventilation, hypoxemia and hypercarbia.[33,34] These agents must be used with caution in sleep apnea patients as the frequency and severity of respiratory events worsen after narcotic administration. Because upper airway reconstructive surgeries may require narcotic agents for 10 to 14 days for adequate pain control,[23] there may be a dilemma between giving adequate pain control and avoiding complications. It has been assumed that narcotic agents administered through IM or IV routes cause more respiratory suppression that those given by an oral route. It is clear that patient-controlled analgesia (via a pump) does not seem to prevent airway-related complications, although the literature is insufficient to evaluate whether or not nurse-administered narcotics are safer than patient-controlled analgesia in OSAHS patients.[2]

In general, however, narcotic agents should be titrated for pain severity and used only when non-narcotic agents are ineffective. Mild to moderate pain can be treated with oral opioid agents (codeine, hydrocodone, oxycodone, or propoxyphene), as these agents appear to have only mild effects on the respiratory system. Non-narcotic options (acetaminophen) or centrally acting agents (tramadol hydrochloride) have no effects on the respiratory system. Nonsteroidal anti-inflammatory agents (ibuprophen, naproxen, and ketolorac tromethamine) or the cyclooxygenase 2 agents (celocoxib) may also be helpful but should be used with caution due to the potential for increased bleeding. Topical anesthetics (benzocaine) are also useful supplements to control pain.

Use of Continuous Positive Airway Pressure and Supplemental Oxygen

Because narcotics and anesthetic agents cause hypoventilation, and microscopic atelectasis causes hypoxemia, supplemental oxygen is typically used after surgery until normal oxygen saturation can be maintained while breathing room air. Severe oxygen desaturation can lead to cardiac arrhythmias, myocardial infarction, or stroke. In sleep apnea patients, the goal is to keep both the waking and sleeping oxygen saturation in a normal range (above 90%). Use of supplemental oxygen does not prevent apneas and hypopneas and may actually reduce awareness of the respiratory events, because there may be no desaturation with shorter apneas or hypopneas. As a result, the preferred approach is to use supplemental oxygen to maintain the waking oxygen saturation, PAP to maintain the sleeping oxygen saturation, and oxygen and PAP for patients with both waking and sleeping hypoxemia.

Except for certain limitations, PAP can be safely used after most upper airway surgeries to prevent respiratory events during sleep[35] and should be used in all patients able to use it before surgery. After surgery, PAP may also reduce the risk of gastroesophageal reflux.[36] Patients should be instructed to bring their own PAP machine to the surgery facility for postoperative use at the preoperative pressure setting. The PAP pressure may be changed, if needed, to a higher pressure in the presence of tissue edema or persistent desaturations during sleep or to a lower pressure if unable to tolerate higher pressures. PAP should not be used after mandibular or maxillary advancement due to the potential of subcutaneous emphysema. After nasal surgery, PAP can still be used with a full face mask instead of a nasal mask or nasal pillows.

Reducing Airway Edema

Upper airway surgery or a difficult intubation may cause airway edema and airway compromise in patients with severe sleep apnea, multiple sites of airway narrowing, or who are undergoing multiple airway surgeries. Tissue edema occurs in all surgeries, even after laser and radiofrequency procedures.[37,38] Administration of systemic steroids reduces edema in the upper airway[39] and, for optimal effect, should be administered before surgery and several times postoperatively. The preferred corticosteroid agent is dexamethasone (10–15 mg every 6–12 hours in adults) as it has the least sodium retention of available steroids.

Soft tissue edema may also be reduced by cooling of the tissue before incision or after surgery. Precooling with ice has been shown to reduce edema in thermal wounds from lasers[39] or cautery units. Application of external ice packs or sucking on ice chips reduces pain and swelling. Antibiotics may also limit edema by reducing bacterial contamination of a surgical wound. Systemic antibiotic prophylaxis given within 1 hour of incision reduces the risk of infection in contaminated oral surgical fields and reduces pain after procedures, such as tonsillectomy. For oropharyngeal surgeries, pre- and postoperative topical chlorhexidine rinses reduces bacterial counts in the oral cavity. Perioperative use of a broad-spectrum antibiotic agent with anaerobic coverage should be considered for sleep apnea patients undergoing any upper airway surgery.

Nasal obstruction and nasal packing worsen sleep apnea[40] and improving the nasal airway can reduce apnea severity.[41] After nasal surgery, it is best to use methods that avoid nasal packing, such as quilting septal sutures, septal splints, nasal tubes, or nasopharyngeal airways sewn into place. A decongestant nasal spray (oxymetazoline) or oral decongestant is also effective in reducing nasal resistance after nasal surgery or nasal intubation.

Postoperative Sedatives

Because of the frequency of insomnia, it is common to prescribe a sedative hypnotic before and after surgery. Sedative hypnotics and anxiolytics, however, should be avoided due to their adverse effects on arousal thresholds, apnea duration and frequency, and oxygen desaturation. If a sleep aid is necessary, there are two short-acting nonbenzodiazepine hypnotic agents that have only a minimal effect on sleep apnea severity. Zaloplon had no significant effect on the apnea/hypopnea index compared with placebo in mild to moderate sleep apnea patients and had no effect on oxygen saturation.[42,43] Zolpidem also had no significant effect on the apnea/hypopnea index in these patients but did reduce the lowest oxygen saturation and the total time with oxygen saturation less than 90% and 80%.[42,43]

Deep Vein Thrombosis Prophylaxis

Obesity, prolonged bed rest, advanced age, and long surgical procedures predispose to deep vein thrombosis (DVT) and pulmonary emboli. The risk of DVT can be reduced by application of sequential compression stockings, elastic stockings, early ambulation, and subcutaneous heparin or enoxaparin sodium. Because many sleep apnea patients are overweight, DVT prophylaxis is indicated for most patients undergoing surgery for sleep apnea.

Blood Pressure Control

Hypertension is more common in OSAHS patients due to increased sympathetic tone, and these patients are at increased risk of postoperative hypertension.[14,15] More than half of OSAHS patients undergoing upper airway surgery require treatment with an antihypertensive agent in the recovery room to maintain a systolic blood pressure below 160 mm Hg and diastolic below 90 mm Hg (Samuel A. Mickelson, MD, unpublished data, 2001). Blood pressure control is especially important after osteotomies, because bleeding from bone is blood pressure dependent and cannot be controlled with ligatures. Elevated blood pressure is important to reduce the risk of postoperative bleeding, hematomas, and secondary tissue edema.

Criteria for Discharge

The literature is insufficient to offer guidance about which criteria must be met before patients are ready to go home. Consultants to the American Society of Anesthesiologists agreed that the room air oxygen saturation should return to its preoperative baseline, that patients should not be hypoxemic or develop airway obstruction when left undisturbed, and that patients should be monitored for 7 hours after the last episode of airway obstruction or hypoxemia while breathing room air in a nonstimulating environment.[2] Unfortunately, these guidelines are not reasonable. Most patients with OSAHS undergo surgery because they will not or cannot use PAP. Because surgery is not instantly curative in most patients, most continue to have apnea after surgery. A more practical recommendation is that the waking oxygen saturation, respiratory event frequency, and degree of hypoxemia are no worse at discharge than at baseline (preoperative sleep study). If there is continued significant sleep apnea or desaturation noted in the hospital, then patients should be discharged with the same edema preventing measures that were used in the hospital (head of bed elevation, decongestants, and so forth) or supplemental oxygen if needed.

Other discharge guidelines should include adequate swallowing to be able to maintain hydration and nutrition and pain controlled with oral analgesics. In addition, patients' vital signs (temperature, pulse, blood pressure, and respiratory rate) should be stable before discharge.

SUMMARY

Sleep apnea patients pose a challenge for surgeons, anesthesiologists, and surgical facility as there is an increased risk for anesthetic and postoperative complications, including airway obstruction, myocardial infarction, stroke, cardiac arrhythmia, and sudden death. Precautions are required before and after surgery to minimize these risks. Screening for sleep apnea should be done for all surgical patients as many patients have not yet been diagnosed. Safe perioperative management requires judicious use of narcotics and sedating medications, reducing upper airway edema, prevention of aspiration and DVT, blood pressure control, use of PAP if possible, and proper postoperative monitoring. Although the literature is lacking for each specific recommendation, the guidelines presented here are based on more than 20 years of experience and are supported by the peer-reviewed medical literature.

REFERENCES

1. Young T, Palta M, Dempsey J, et al. The occurrence of sleep-disordered breathing among middle–aged adults. N Engl J Med 1993;328:1230–5.
2. American Society of Anesthesiologists. Practice guidelines for the perioperative management of patients with obstructive sleep apnea. A report by the American Society of Anesthesiologists Task Force on Perioperative Management of Patients with Obstructive Sleep Apnea. Anesthesiology 2006;104:1081–93.
3. Aurell J, Elmqvist D. Sleep in the surgical intensive care unit: continuous polygraphic recording of nine patients receiving postoperative care. Br Med J 1985;290:1029–32.
4. Rosenberg J, Rosenberg-Adamsen S, Kehlet H. Post-operative sleep disturbances: causes, factors and effects on outcome. Eur J Anaesthesiol 1995; 10(Suppl):28–30.
5. Cullen DJ. Obstructive sleep apnea and postoperative analgesia—a potentially dangerous combination. J Clin Anesth 2001;13:83–5.
6. Fairbanks DNF. Uvulopalatopharyngoplasty complications and avoidance strategies. Otolaryngol Head Neck Surg 1990;102:239–45.
7. Bonara M, St John WM, Bledsoe TA. Differential elevation by protriptyline and depression by diazepam of upper airway motor activity. Am Rev Respir Dis 1985;131:41–5.
8. Guilleminault C, Silvestri R, Mondini S, et al. Aging and sleep apnea: action of benzodiazipine, acetozolamide, alcohol and sleep deprivation in a healthy elderly group. J Gerontol 1984;39: 655–66.
9. Berry RB, Kouchi K, Bower J, et al. Triazolam in patients with obstructive sleep apnea. Am J Respir Crit Care Med 1995;151:450–4.
10. DeMeester TR, Johnson LF, Joseph GJ, et al. Patterns of gastroesophageal reflux in health and disease. Ann Surg 1976;184:459–70.
11. Mercer CD, Wren SF, DaCosta LR, et al. Lower esophageal sphincter pressure and gastroesophageal pressure gradients in excessively obese patients. J Med 1987;18:135–46.
12. Vaughan RW, Bauer S, Wise L. Volume and PH of gastric juice in obese patients. Anesthesiology 1975;43:686–9.
13. Warwick JP, Mason DG. Obstructive sleep apnoea in children. Anaesthesia 1998;53:571–9.
14. Worsnop CJ, Pierce RJ, Naughton M. Systemic hypertension and obstructive sleep apnea. Sleep 1993;16:S148–9.
15. Bonsignore MR, Marrone O, Insalaco G, et al. The cardiovascular effects of obstructive sleep apnoeas: analysis of pathogenic mechanisms. Eur Respir J 1994;7:786–805.
16. Benumof JL. Management of the difficult airway. Anesthesiology 1991;75:1087–110.
17. American Society of Anesthesiologists. Practice guidelines for management of the difficult airway. A report by the American Society of Anesthesiologists Task Force on Management of the Difficult Airway. Anesthesiology 1993;78:597–602.
18. Benumof JL. Laryngeal mask airway and the ASA difficult airway algorithm. Anesthesiology 1996;84: 686–99.
19. Mickelson SA. Upper airway bypass surgery for obstructive sleep apnea syndrome. Otolaryngol Clin North Am 1996;31(6):1013–23.
20. Meoli AL, Rosen CL, Kristo D, et al. Report of the AASM clinical practice review committee. Upper airway management of the adult patient with obstructive sleep apnea in the perioperative perod—avoiding complications. Sleep 2003;26(8): 1060–5.
21. Berry RB, Kouchi KG, Bower JL, et al. Effect of upper airway anesthesia on obstructive sleep apnea. Am J Respir Crit Care Med 1995;151: 1857–61.
22. Johnson JT, Sanders MH. Breathing during sleep immediately after uvulopalatopharyngoplasty. Laryngoscope 1986;96:1236–8.
23. Troell RJ, Powell NB, Riley TW, et al. Comparison of postoperative pain between laser assisted uvulopalatoplasty, uvulopalatopharyngoplasty, and radiofrequency volumetric tissue reduction of the palate. Otolaryngol Head Neck Surg 2000;122:402–9.
24. Rosenberg J, Rasmussen GI, Wojdemann KR, et al. Ventilatory pattern and associated episodic hypoxaemia in the late postoperative period in the general surgical ward. Anaesthesia 1999;54: 323–8.
25. Knill RL, Moote CA, Skinner MI, et al. Anesthesia with abdominal surgery leads to intense REM sleep during the first postoperative week. Anesthesiology 1990;73:52–61.
26. Sanders MH, Johnson JT, Keller FA, et al. The acute effects of uvulopalatopharyngoplasty on breathing during sleep in sleep apnea patients. Sleep 1988; 11:75–89.
27. Esclamado RM, Gleen MG, McCulloch TM, et al. Perioperative complications and risk factors in the surgical treatment of obstructive sleep apnea syndrome. Laryngoscope 1989;99:1125–9.
28. Haavisto L, Suonpaa J. Complications of uvulopalatopharyngoplasty. Clin Otolaryngol 1994;9: 243–7.
29. Macaluso RA, Reams C, Vrabec DP, et al. Uvulopalatopharyngoplasty: post-operative management

and evaluation of results. Ann Otol Rhinol Laryngol 1989;98:502–7.

30. Hathaway B, Johnson JT. Safety of uvulopalatopharyngoplasty as outpatient surgery. Otolaryngol Head Neck Surg 2006;134(4):542–4.

31. Kezirian EJ, Weaver EM, Yueh B, et al. Incidence of serious complications after uvulopalatopharyngoplasty. Laryngoscope 2004;114(3):450–3.

32. Mickelson SA, Hakim I. Is post operative intensive care monitoring necessary after uvulopalatopharyngoplasty? Otolaryngol Head Neck Surg 1998; 119(4):352–6.

33. Mickelson SA. Perioperative and anesthesia management in obstructive sleep apnea surgery. In: Fairbanks DNF, Mickelson SA, Woodson BT, editors. Snoring and obstructive sleep apnea. 3rd edition. Philadelphia: Lippencott Williams & Wilkins; 2003. p. 223–32.

34. Bailey PL, Egan TD, Stanley TH. Intravenous opioid anesthetics. In: Miller RD, editor. Anesthesia. 5th edition. Philadelphia: Churchill Livingstone; 2000. p. 273–376.

35. Powell NB, Riley RW, Guilleminault C, et al. Obstructive sleep apnea, continuous positive airway pressure, and surgery. Otolaryngol Head Neck Surg 1988;99(4):362–9.

36. Kerr P, Shoenut JP, Millar J, et al. Nasal CPAP reduces gastroesophageal reflux in obstructive sleep apnea syndrome. Chest 1992;101(6):1539–44.

37. Terris DJ, Clerk AA, Norbash AM, et al. Characterization of postoperative edema following laser-assisted uvulopalatoplasty using MRI and polysomnography: implications for the outpatient treatment of obstructive sleep apnea syndrome. Laryngoscope 1996;106:124–8.

38. Powell NB, Riley RW, Troell RJ, et al. Radiofrequency volumetric reduction of the tongue. A porcine pilot study for the treatment of obstructive sleep apnea syndrome. Chest 1997;111:1348–55.

39. Sheppard LM, Werkhaven JA, Mickelson SA. The effect of steroids or tissue pre-cooling on edema and tissue thermal coagulation after CO_2 laser impact. Lasers Surg Med 1992;12:137–46.

40. Olsen KD. The nose and its impact on snoring and obstructive sleep apnea. In: Fairbanks DNF, editor. Snoring and obstructive sleep apnea. New York: Raven Press; 1987. p. 199–226.

41. Dayall VS, Phillipson EA. Nasal surgery in the management of sleep apnea. Ann Otol Rhinol Laryngol 1985;94:550–4.

42. George CFP. Perspectives on the management of insomnia in patients with chronic respiratory disorders. Sleep 2000;23(Suppl 1):S31–5.

43. Mickelson SA. Avoidance of complications in sleep apnea patients. In: Terris DJ, Goode RL, editors. Surgical management of sleep apnea and snoring. Boca Raton (FL): Taylor & Francis Group; 2005. p. 453–64.

Reconstruction of Airway Soft Tissues in Obstructive Sleep Apnea

B. Tucker Woodson, MD*, Peter D. O'Connor, MD, OD

KEYWORDS

- Obstructive sleep apnea • Palatopharyngoplasty
- Glossectomy • Nasal surgery snoring • Adenotonsillectomy

Surgery for obstructive sleep apnea (OSA) is multimodal. Procedures and aims of treatment vary. Surgery, medical devices, and medical therapy each may contribute to individualized patient care. There is no single procedure or intervention that "cures" upper airway obstruction. Treatment varies as the disease varies. In addition, surgical treatment varies because the level of obstruction and influence on air flow occurs at multiple levels and from many structures.

Simply put, the problem in OSA centers on an airway too small for a given individual's physiology. The human larynx, unlike other mammals, has a more caudal location, away from the skull base. The result is a conduit prone to collapse and obstruct where there is soft tissue. Portions of the upper airway from the nasal tip to the glottis are surrounded by osseous or cartilaginous structures that provide some stability. The remainder of the airway is composed of soft tissue.

The flow of air through a collapsible tube is influenced by the difference in upstream, downstream, and intraluminal forces (as a Starling resistor). Multiple levels of the upper airway influence obstruction. The propensity for collapse at each level may be influenced by various tissues including muscle, mucosa, vascular tissue, and mechanoreceptors. Our understanding of how each of these components participates in the obstruction is incomplete. Despite this, for some individuals, surgery can play a critical role as part of the multimodal algorithm for treating OSA.[1,2]

The concept of surgery for sleep-disordered breathing is often misunderstood. It is not a unique procedure, or even set of procedures, but a reconstructive approach to improve airway form and function with the goal of reducing severity of disease. With this concept the goal of surgery is not limited to surgery as a first-line "cure" of all disease but rather a tool used also for ancillary treatment combined with other medical modalities or as salvage. Although surgical salvage treatment after medical failure is an important role for the surgeon it is not the only and may not be the primary one.

Criticism of surgery for sleep apnea and sleep-disordered breathing is often enthusiastic because in major reviews, procedures are pooled, treating all techniques as equivalent. Further, many fail to account or understand that multiple levels of the airway and therefore multiple structures may be involved. Last, assessing clinical outcomes when multiple interventions or procedures are needed especially for surgery is difficult. This article is not intended as a critical assessment of surgical outcomes but rather will focus on airway structures and the nature of the procedures applied to influence them.

STRUCTURE

A hurdle impeding the progress of surgical treatment of OSA and sleep-disordered breathing is the concept that surgery treats the soft tissues around the airway. This focus on the "donut" or the soft tissue and skeletal ring surrounding the airway distracts attention from the "donut hole." The airway lumen is the ultimate literal and

Division of Sleep Medicine, Department of Otolaryngology and Communication Sciences, Medical College of Wisconsin, 9200 W. Wisconsin Avenue, Milwaukee, WI 53226, USA
* Corresponding author.
E-mail address: bwoodson@mcw.edu (B.T. Woodson).

Oral Maxillofacial Surg Clin N Am 21 (2009) 435–445
doi:10.1016/j.coms.2009.08.005

oralmaxsurgery.theclinics.com

figurative pathway of disease. Obviously, tissue defines a lumen, but it is the nature and function of the lumen that is pathologic in most patients, not the tissues themselves. A tissue focus may, in some ways, perpetuate the widespread impression that there may be a single common method or procedure to treat the disorder. With this concept, all that is needed to fix sleep apnea is for someone to discover the secret procedure. Although appealing, because of its simplicity, the concept fails in most patients because it is not the "palate" that is abnormal but the associated "palatal airway." The key outcome of "reconstructive airway" surgery is normalization of airflow and not normalization of tissue. Unfortunately, airflow, especially in the upper airway, is complex and there are few uncomplicated solutions. OSA is not just a structural disease but also involves a loss of physiologic compensation; however, a reconstructive approach may provide marked clinical improvement when applied appropriately.

Reconstructive surgery has the goal of improving form and function. Tissues may be moved, removed, or remodeled using many techniques. In the airway, acute goals include changing airway size, volume, shape, and compliance. This must be achieved while limiting morbidity or negative alteration of other functions of the upper airway, including smell, taste, swallowing, and speech. Interventions for the upper airway are still evolving, and many new ones are being assessed. Many techniques used in the past will likely be abandoned.

Current methods are stages of an evolutionary process and certainly will change. The two surgical approaches to treat OSA and related disorders include bypassing the upper airway, or reconstructing the skeletal or soft tissues. A large variety of techniques have been described, reflecting, to some degree, surgeon preferences but also the wide variability of upper airway structural anatomy that contributes to disease. The skeletal and cartilage framework not only determines much of the size, shape, and compliance of the airway but also describes the intrinsic patterns of facial growth that correlate to risk factors for sleep-disordered breathing. The position of the human larynx in the neck instead of at the skull base is important. This position is speculated to be related to changes in human cranial development and growth patterns. Cranial development, therefore, can affect both facial and airway form. A major risk factor for OSA is a longer soft tissue pharyngeal airway superior to the larynx. This structure is more susceptible to collapse from changes in body position, vascular volume, and tissue edema, and loss of muscle tone during sleep. Skull base

development in OSA also creates a narrowed posterior maxillary airspace.

Soft tissue changes worsen an airway already at risk. Often, a constellation of abnormalities are markers of facial skeletal abnormalities in OSA. These may include increased distance of the hyoid bone from the mandibular plane, decreased mandibular and maxillary projection, increased vertical length of the lower anterior face, increased vertical length of the posterior airway, and increased cervical angulation. In addition, other factors contribute to OSA.

Facial structure interacts with obesity to create apnea risk. In the Wisconsin Sleep Cohort, a population-based study, two thirds of the apnea-hypopnea index (AHI) was explained by a combination of facial structure and obesity.[3] In nonobese subjects, facial structure alone explains AHI. Individuals with normal craniofacial structures require morbid obesity or other airway pathology to display OSA. Soft tissues are frequently abnormal in OSA, both primarily and also as a consequence of the disease.

There is a strong familial aggregation of apnea, and in some populations, this has been linked to soft tissue abnormalities. Genetic studies have demonstrated the inheritability of abnormal lateral wall size and tongue size in populations of patients with apnea.[4] Soft tissue abnormalities include a longer and wider soft palate, larger tongue, smaller oropalatal airspace, a posteriorly placed epiglottis, and smaller posterior airspace.

Obesity alters OSA in both direct and indirect ways. It increases the severity of OSA by worsening hypoxemia during sleep. Obesity also effects metabolism, ventilation, and lung volume to worsen apnea. Leptin and other inflammatory obesity-related cytokines may increase CO_2 response, and central ventilatory sensitivity augments the tendency toward periodic breathing and increased airway instability. Increased soft tissue tongue size has also been associated with obesity. Fat distribution around the neck has long been postulated, without evidence, to compromise the airway.

ANESTHETIC CONSIDERATIONS

Patients with sleep apnea may have unique preoperative, intraoperative, and postoperative care issues.[5] Difficulty with intubation and extubation related to facial structural or ventilatory control issues exist. High-risk patients include, but are not limited to, patients with severe obesity, poor pulmonary reserve, pharyngeal tissue redundancy, hypoxemia, access to narcotic use, multiple airway surgical procedures, and excessive sleepiness. Controversy exists as to the appropriateness of outpatient surgery and the need for intensive postoperative monitoring.[6] Postoperative management can be helped in many cases with the use of nasal continuous positive airway pressure (CPAP). Rarely, tracheotomy is required. Objective monitoring to include pulse oximetry has been advocated; however, it is critical to realize that oximetry does not measure hypoventilation, especially when assessed on an intermittent basis or when low-flow oxygen is in use. Close nursing observation is necessary in the perioperative period. Symptoms of respiratory insufficiency and hypercarbia may include increased pulse and respiratory rate, elevated blood pressure, and agitation or restlessness. Studies suggest that the stimulating and disruptive environments of the hospital provide a degree of safety and that risk may increase in quiet and unobserved areas. Risk increases with sedation, dehydration (increasing tenacious secretions), and increased doses of narcotics. Postoperative interventions for patients with apnea who have airway and nonairway surgery may include treating nasal airways, nasal CPAP, patient positioning (elevation of the head of bed), adequate hydration, corticosteroids, and other non-narcotic pain medication. Patients with sleep apnea are also at elevated risk because of significant comorbidities of hypertension, cardiac and pulmonary disease, and obesity.

AIRWAY ASSESSMENT

Airway assessment in patients at risk for OSA may include (1) identifying features that predict risk of apnea and severity of disease; (2) improving patient selection with the goal of eliminating patients at high risk of failure; and (3) identifying specific structural abnormalities to direct reconstruction. Assessment must also balance the severity of the disorder, host comorbid conditions, and anticipate clinical outcomes to determine surgical approach. Patients, especially those with high risk factors for disease and unfavorable airway structure who are unable or unwilling to proceed with limited interventions, may warrant approaches such as maxillomandibular surgery or tracheotomy.

Methods of evaluation include physical examination, endoscopy, and radiologic assessment. Inspection without instrumentation provides information about facial growth (hyoid, neck, mandible, and maxillary positioning). Significant nasal disease can be identified or suspected with limited instruments. Routine physical examination may assess the nasal valve, septal position, high arched palate, tonsil size, tongue size, and evidence of pharyngeal tissue damage. All patients deserve an adequate examination, especially if initial therapy is less than completely successful.

FRIEDMAN STAGING

The Friedman staging system for the oral cavity and oropharyngeal portions of the upper airway defines four stages based on the following: (1) tonsil size (1 to 4+); (2) a modification of the Mallampati classification (1 to 4+); (3) presence or absence of severe obesity (> or < BMI of 40 kg/m^2); and (4) major craniofacial abnormalities.[7] The Friedman staging system identifies patients at risk for apnea who present with symptoms of snoring. It also demonstrates both positive and negative uvulopalatopharyngoplasty (UPPP) predictive values.

Friedman staging groups tonsil size as "favorable" (tonsil grades 3 and 4, ie, large tonsils), or "unfavorable" (tonsil grades 1 and 2, ie, small tonsils). The Modified Mallampati classification is "favorable" (grades 1 and 2, visualizing the free margin of the soft palate), and "unfavorable" (grades 3 and 4, free margin of palate not visible) on examination. Friedman Stage I has demonstrated high success rates with limited palatal surgery alone. Friedman Stage III demonstrates less success rate with limited palatal surgery.

TRACHEOTOMY

Historically, tracheotomy was the first intervention for severe OSA. The procedure has high social morbidity. Long-term studies demonstrate that, although tracheotomy reduces the morbidity and mortality associated with sleep apnea, it has primary morbidity as well.[8] Obesity, a short neck, a low larynx, and the inability to extend the neck may complicate tracheotomy. Experienced centers often perform "skin-flap" tracheotomy techniques that reduce associated morbidity. In OSA, the airway in wakefulness is patent, and tracheotomies may be occluded during wakefulness and opened only during sleep. In perceived psychosocial implications, risks of stenosis, infection, and other potential complications, tracheotomy has limited application. With the advent of acceptable medical treatment options, tracheotomy is often reserved for severe disease, complicated airway management, perioperative airway safety, and for patients too ill for other procedures or therapies.

NASAL SURGERY

A seeming paradox has been described regarding the nose and OSA. Nasal obstruction has clearly been demonstrated as a risk factor for OSA, yet treatment does not necessarily affect the disease risk. Aside from the extraordinarily unlikely possibility that nasal disease does not impact sleep treatment, studies must be interpreted correctly. Symptomatic nasal obstruction is poorly associated with abnormal resistance, so diagnosis of structural nasal disease is difficult.

Nasal airway disease is predominantly in the nasal valve, which contributes 70% of upper airway resistance in adult humans. The nasal septum is only a limited contributor, yet all surgical treatment studies base conclusions on interventions overwhelmingly limited to septoplasty. Furthermore, as a secondary risk factor, measuring nasal obstruction independently of the primary risk factors introduces confounding variability. This makes it difficult to measure outcomes unless the primary risk factors also have been controlled. To our best knowledge, no studies have done this to date. Last, and most important, a patent and open nasal airway is important for sleep and sleep quality.[9,10] Using a metric such as AHI is potentially incorrect. Data show support that a patent nasal airway is a major predictor of successful medical and surgical treatment. Treating an abnormal nasal airway is important in effectively treating sleep-disordered breathing,[11] but this requires accurate diagnosis and an understanding of comprehensive treatment methods.

As noted previously in humans, progressive shortening of the nasal maxillary complex and elongation of the pharyngeal airway is a common theme in facial growth and development. A smaller maxilla narrows the retromaxillary space but also markedly reduces the volume of the nasal cavity. The abnormality in the nose may not be deviation or tissue hypertrophy but, ultimately, a predisposed small nasal cavity. Improvements in nasal obstruction after maxillary expansion have been reported.[12,13]

Nasal obstruction demonstrates greater positional dependence and increased obstruction in patients with OSA compared with normal subjects. The cause of this is unresolved but may result from structural and physiologic medical disorders, including vasomotor instability and increased inflammation. Nasal blockage may (1) reduce nasal afferent reflexes, which help maintain muscular tone of the upper airway; (2) augment the tendency for mouth opening, which destabilizes the lower pharyngeal airway (by posterior rotation, vertical opening, and inferior displacement of the hyoid); (3) reduce humidification, increase mucus viscosity, and increase surface tension forces; and (4) increase upstream airway resistance predisposing to downstream airway collapse.

Treating nasal obstruction may have a significant impact on snoring, OSA, central sleep apnea, and insomnia. Physiologically, treatment reduces airway resistance, reduces work of breathing, decreases ventilatory effort and arousal, and decreases cyclic breathing instability. Treatment varies according to pathologic findings and may include correction of septal deviations, inferior turbinate hypertrophy, nasal valve collapse, or removal of nasal polyps. Treatment of nasal obstruction improves daytime and nighttime subjective quality of life, sleep, and daytime performance. Controversy exists as to the safety of performing simultaneous nasal and other pharyngeal surgeries. Which sleep apnea surgeries are safe to pursue combined with nasal surgery has not been established. Criteria to consider include but are not limited to the following: (1) mild OSA; (2) no anticipated requirement of nasal packing that would preclude perioperative nasal CPAP; (3) no major medical comorbidity that will place the patient at risk (hypertension, coronary artery disease, or other vascular disease); and (4) appropriate and skilled postoperative monitoring and observation.

TONSILLECTOMY/ADENOIDECTOMY (ADULTS)

In adults, removal of nonhypertrophic palatine tonsils is generally ineffective as an isolated procedure for treating OSA. However, removal of nonhypertrophic tonsils is commonly done as a part of other pharyngoplasty procedures. Adults with enlarged tonsils, without other major airway abnormalities, and without profound morbid obesity may respond to tonsillectomy. Adenoidal enlargement in adults is uncommon and, if present, warrants referral for a causative etiology, viral infection, systemic disease, or neoplasm.

TONSILLECTOMY/ADENOIDECTOMY (PEDIATRICS)

Adenotonsillectomy is the treatment of choice for OSA in children. Traditionally, it has been considered highly effective but its actual effectiveness is uncertain. In pediatric patients with uncomplicated disease, a meta-analysis of level 4 evidence (case series) demonstrated that tonsillectomy and adenoidectomy reduced the AHI by an average of 13.9 events per hour and normalized AHI in approximately 80% of patients.[14] Outcomes vary by population and are affected by airway and facial structure, obesity, nasal pathologic findings, allergies, and underlying medical conditions. Factors predictive of elevated AHI postoperatively in noncomplicated pediatric patients include enlarged inferior turbinates, deviated nasal septum, Mallampati scores of 3 and 4, and retropositioned mandibles. Persistent airway inflammatory disease has been identified in other groups and responds successfully to anti-inflammatory therapies, including topical nasal steroids and leukotriene inhibitors.[15]

Adenotonsillectomy has demonstrated significant improvements in behavior and school performance independent of final AHI levels.[16–18] Quality-of-life measures have been shown to improve despite the level of disease and can be maintained after surgery.[17,19,20]

Pediatric patients with sleep apnea may represent an at-risk population for sleep apnea independent of hypertrophic tonsils and adenoids. Associated problems include obesity and disproportionate facial growth and development. Identifying children at risk of persistent apnea and additional treatment may be critical. A family history of sleep apnea associated with findings of a high arched palate, long faces, or retrognathic mandible may warrant orthodontic assessment and treatment in addition to tonsil and adenoid surgery. Appropriate treatment of the nose also is important in children and should not be overlooked. This may include addressing hypertrophied turbinates, a deviated septum, or the maxillary foundation. Recent data highlight the importance of looking at multiple levels and structures in children with OSA.[21–23] The combination of adenotonsillectomy and orthodontic expansion may be necessary for some patients to achieve successful treatment.

PALATOPHARYNGOPLASTY

UPPP was first described by Fujita.[24] The procedure removes the distal soft palate, faucial tonsils, uvula, and redundant mucosa from the anterior and posterior tonsillar pillars. The posterior pillar is then sutured anteriorly and the mucosa approximated. Multiple variations of the technique have been described. Its effectiveness for sleep apnea is not related to symptomatic reduction in snoring, but instead is associated with increases in pharyngeal airway size in the retropalatal airway segment. UPPP is generally combined with other surgical procedures to treat other airway sites. The procedure may be contraindicated in patients with velopharyngeal insufficiency (VPI), submucous cleft palate, a nonpalatal level of obstruction, and in patients whose speech or swallowing may be at special risk. Aggressive resection of the palate with UPPP techniques has demonstrated no improvement in success, but does increase the risk of VPI. Side effects of UPPP are common and include mucosal dryness, sensation of oropharyngeal tightness or phlegm, pharyngeal dysphagia, and severe postoperative pain. Major complications are rare and include acute respiratory distress, VPI, rhinolalia, nasopharyngeal stenosis, and hemorrhage. Respiratory distress and fatality with UPPP are rare.

Controlled and randomized studies for sleep apnea surgery are exceedingly difficult to perform. However, such studies have been performed and do demonstrate UPPP is effective in treating physiologic measures of sleep and respiration, quality of life, risk of motor vehicle accidents, cardiovascular risks, and mortality.[23] The effectiveness of palate surgical procedures varies. Not all techniques are equivalent. Using the Friedman staging system, outcomes can be better stratified (Friedman stage 1 = 70% success, stage 2 = 40% success, and stage 3 = 10% success). Traditional UPPP is most useful in individuals with massive tissue redundancy of the pharynx that requires excision and enlarged tonsils. Avoidance of excessive removal of the distal soft palate is important to prevent incompetence between the soft palate and tongue and worsening possible nasal CPAP tolerance by increasing the potential for a mouth leak. Data demonstrate that failure of UPPP often is attributable to persistent obstruction at the retropalatal airway segment, not just obstruction in the lower pharynx, as has been often assumed.

Several methods of UPPP have now been described and compared. These techniques reconstruct the soft and hard tissue framework of the palate and not only modify the mucosa and tonsils. Described techniques include lateral pharyngoplasty and expansion sphincteroplasty. Lateral pharyngoplasty exposes and plicates the lateral pharyngeal wall muscles and superior constrictor proximal toward the hamulus to the free margin of the soft palate.[24,25] Expansion sphincteroplasty exposes, isolates, and divides the palatopharyngeus muscle on the pharyngeal wall and uses this muscle as a sling to advance and open the soft palate and pharynx (**Fig. 1**).[26] An additional technique to address obstruction by the soft palate is palatal advancement. Palatal advancement removes distal hard palate to advance the soft palate anteriorly and superiorly and appears to be most beneficial in certain patients with retropalatal obstruction (**Fig. 2**).[27] We have found that in some patients, these techniques can have significant effect in improving

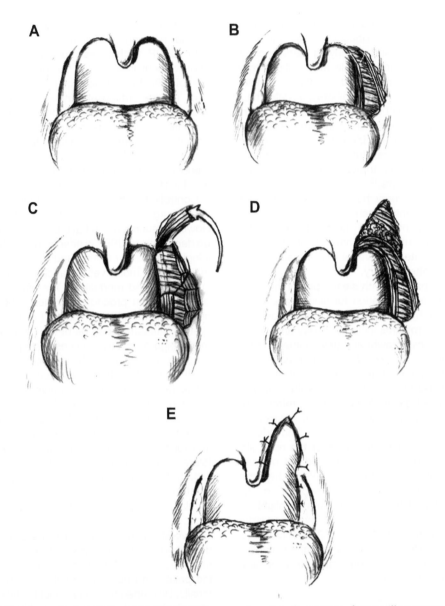

Fig. 1. Lateral pharyngoplasty is depicted. Steps for the procedure include exposure for tonsillectomy, palatopharyngoplasty (*A*). Tonsillectomy is performed preserving muscle and all mucosa (*B*). A portion of the palatopharyngeous muscle is carefully dissected from the constrictor muscle and from the medial mucosa. The muscle is elevated proximally to the approximate level of the soft palate (*C*). It is then rotated approximately 110 degrees anteriorly, laterally, and superiorly and sutured to fascia in the area of the hamulus (*D*). A dorsal palatal flap closure is shown (*E*).

the size of the "donut hole" without removing any tissue in some cases but rather reconstructing the tissues that are present.

SNORING

Multiple palate procedures have been advocated to treat primary snoring. Most have shown short-term effectiveness.[28] Primary snoring is not an isolated disorder and may represent a benign point in time of a progressive upper airway disease, so conservative treatments with the least side effects and complications should be considered first, if possible.[29] Snoring may be primary palatal or arise from other areas of the pharynx. Furthermore, the etiology of the snoring can be flow restriction at the same site or elsewhere in the airway. As a result, some procedures may

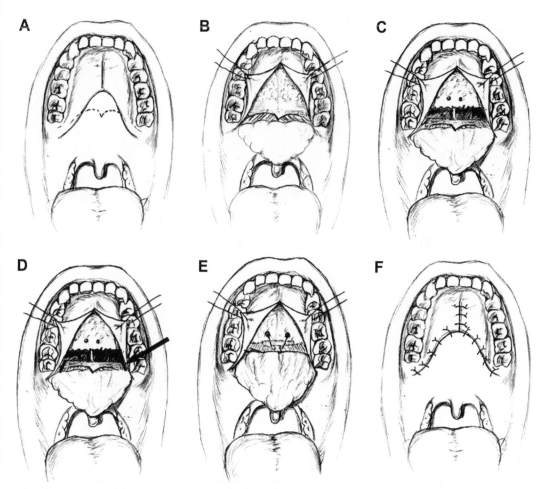

Fig. 2. Steps of palatal advancement are shown. Incisions for palatal flap are shown and allow exposure of the distal hard palate and medial to the greater palatine foramen (*A*). Two lateral flaps and a posterior flap are elevated (*B*). An osteotomy is performed and 8 to 10 mm of distal palate is removed with preservation of mucosa. More proximal through and through drill holes for later suture placement are also performed (*C*). Nasal mucosa is incised as are the tensor tendon medial to the hamulus. This allows mobilization of the soft palate (*D*). The soft palate and osteotomized segment are pulled anteriorly and attached (*E*). Flaps are closed with preservation of all mucosa. Occasionally a small amount of soft tissue debulking of the posterior flap may be helpful (*F*).

not address the source of flow restriction but may change the dynamics of tissue flutter and quality of sound emitted from the tissue.

Laser-assisted uvulopalatoplasty (LAUP) incorporates CO2 laser-enabled hemostatic surgery of the palate under local anesthesia.[30] The palate, velum, and uvula could be resected with healing by secondary intent. Two vertical trenches in the soft palate, lateral to the uvula, of variable width and length at free margin of the distal soft palate are created and the uvula reduced. Surgery may be single stage or "titrated" to improve snoring or the appearance of velopharyngeal dysfunction. LAUP is associated with severe pain and common complaints of pharyngeal dryness.

Serious complications are infrequent. Palatal scarring initially increases tension and reduces snoring, but long-term data (5 years) suggest recurrence of snoring is common. Airway narrowing may occur and worsen sleep apnea. LAUP has not been effective for sleep apnea in clinical trials.[31] Alternatives to the use of lasers also have been described.[32,33] Various less expensive cutting and ablational tools have been used to shorten the palate, remove mucosa, and reduce the uvula and direct healing by secondary intension. All of these tools likely create scar and reduce snoring with variable effectiveness. Failure may be from persistent flow limitation, softening of scar, or flutter at nonpalatal airway sites. All

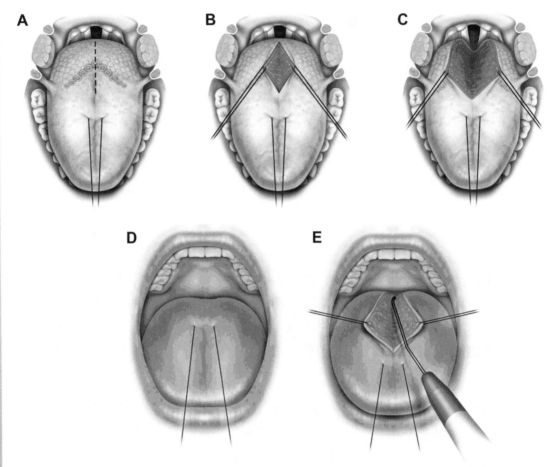

Fig. 3. A method of posterior midline glossectomy is depicted (*A–E*). A traction suture is placed, the location of midline incision is marked, and relative position of the lingual artery and the dorsum of the tongue is identified using ultrasound (*A*). The midline incision deepened and widened and carried back towards the valecula (*B* and *C*). Closure is shown (*D*).

patients, following snoring surgeries, should be cautioned about the risk of recurrence of snoring and the possible later development of overt sleep apnea.

To avoid the extensive thermal damage created to all three layers of the soft palate, as well as chronic inflammation, ulceration, and loss of sero-mucinous glands, alternative approaches to create palatal stiffening have been developed. Techniques using ablational radiofrequency result in less pain in the treatment of snoring compared with laser.[34] Sclerotherapy agents are used to create scar in the mucosa of the soft palate and treat primary snoring.[35] Agents are injected into the submucosa of the soft palate creating scar and tissue slough. The procedure has less pain than laser, and long-term results for snoring are better than 70%, with few major complications. Alternatively, palatal implants have been developed and demonstrate effectiveness for the treatment of primary snoring in selected populations.[36,37]

BASE OF TONGUE TECHNIQUES

Hypopharyngeal techniques include partial glossectomy, ablational glossectomy, mandibular advancement, limited mandibular osteotomies, tongue suspension,[38,39] hyoid suspension, lingual tonsillectomy, and supraglottoplasty. Some evidence-based medicine is available.[40] Ablational radiofrequency of the tongue base can be performed in the office-based setting under local anesthesia, either alone or in combination with other pharyngeal procedures. Complications, including tongue abscess, infection (cellulitis), tongue weakness, changes in speech and swallowing, and acute airway obstruction and edema, are rare. Both studies that are randomized, blinded, and controlled, as well as studies that are uncontrolled have demonstrated effectiveness in reducing the severity and improving the disease-specific quality of life. Effectiveness also has been demonstrated in longer-term studies. These procedures are usually not used independently to definitively treat OSA but are combined with other procedures that reconstruct other segments of the upper airway.

Lingual tonsillar hypertrophy may cause or contribute to sleep apnea. If a patient's tonsils are enlarged, removal may have a marked effect on both sleep and apnea. Historically, difficult exposure and removal of tonsils in patients with sleep apnea, caused by structurally small underlying anatomy and concerns about airway edema, bleeding, and pain, made the threshold to remove these tonsils high. Only in more severe cases was it considered. Newer surgical techniques combining endoscopes and excisional radiofrequency allow easier removal of lingual tonsil tissue. This reduces the threshold of removal and provides a lower morbidity method of enlarging the hypopharyngeal airway when lingual tonsils are present.

Glossectomy may treat lower pharyngeal disease by modifying the shape and size of the soft tissue tongue base, hypopharynx, and supraglottic tissues. Multilevel procedures can also be done.[41,42] Early simple glossectomy procedures improved severe OSA, allowing tracheotomy decannulation. Nonetheless, with the advent of nasal CPAP, the morbidity of major tongue base resections relegated glossectomy to a limited population of patients who were not candidates for other procedures. Midline glossectomy and lingualplasty are partial glossectomies to enlarge the lower pharyngeal airway and treat OSA. In severe obstructive sleep apnea syndrome (OSAS), following UPPP failure, lingualplasty reduces AHI to fewer than 20 events per hour in 70% of patients.[43] Many studies predate the wide application of "evidence-based medicine." Using laser, complication rates approach 25% and include bleeding, severe odynophagia, tongue edema, and taste changes. For this reason, more aggressive glossectomy techniques have not been commonly performed. These procedures directly involve the airway in patients with preexisting airway risk, so the risk was considered high, and a perioperative tracheotomy was historically often performed, resulting in major morbidity for the procedure.

Chabolle and colleagues[44] reported hyoepiglottoplasty using a cervical approach to reduce tongue base size and to reposition the hyolingual complex. Patients were selected based on having soft tissue abnormalities of the pharynx (defined by an abnormal soft tissue hyolaryngeal complex on lateral cephalometric radiographs) and not having craniofacial abnormalities (sella-nasion-subspinale angle <79, and sella-nasion-supramentale angle <77). Glossectomy is performed under a direct vision following a suprahyoid pharyngotomy, with isolation and identification of the hypoglossal nerves and lingual arteries. Partial glossectomy is performed medial to the tonsilar folds and posterior to the circumvallate papillae. Average tongue base reduction was 24 cm^3. Following glossectomy, the hyoid and epiglottis are suspended anteriorly to the mandible. An 80% success rate was reported in 10 consecutive patients. Short-term complications were high (50%) as a result of infection and patients required tracheotomy. Both precluded widespread use. The procedure supports that effective tissue reduction can be an effective treatment. Newer technologies have been described that allow staged glossectomy using endoscopic techniques.[45] Plasma surgical excision allows glossectomy under local or general anesthesia and does not require tracheotomy. The procedure can be performed as outpatient surgery in select patients (**Fig. 3**).

Hyoid movement may stabilize the hypopharyngeal airway including the epiglottis. The hyoid may be suspended anteriorly and superiorly to the mandible or anteriorly and inferiorly to the thyroid cartilage. Hyoid myotomy may be performed with other surgeries such as UPPP or genioglossal advancement.[46,47] Hyoid myotomy is performed transcervically via a neck skin incision. Fascia lata or suture may be used for mandibular suspension. Thyrohyoid suspension has been described with suture or wire. Alternatively, hyomandibular suspension creates a vector of pull that is perhaps more favorable to repositioning the epiglottis and vallecular tongue base, expanding the hypopharyngeal airway lumen. Controlled studies are lacking.

EPIGLOTTIDECTOMY

Removal of the epiglottis has been performed with both midline glossectomy and lingualplasty. In both adults and children, removal of an abnormal epiglottis has improved OSA and upper airway obstruction.[48] Partial resection of the epiglottis with a CO_2 laser has been described as a safe procedure in adults.

SUMMARY

Surgery for obstructive sleep apnea is part of a multimodal algorithm that includes medical therapy. Influences on the flow of air through the lumen of the upper airway can be from a variety of structures and different levels. Various surgical techniques have been developed focusing on modifying either the skeletal anatomy or the soft tissue structures of the upper airway. Reconstructive airway surgery focuses on normalizing airflow while limiting morbidity and other functions of the upper airway.

Successful outcomes for any surgery can be dependent on several factors. A primary factor is understanding the intended goal of the procedure. In patients with sleep apnea, a specific surgery is rarely intended to be curative but rather ancillary to other methods of therapy. However, some procedures have been shown to independently improve quality of life as well as the acceptance of medical therapy. Additional factors that influence outcomes include choosing the correct procedure and the proper execution of the technique. Airflow in obstructive sleep apnea is influenced by multiple levels. It is important to understand that some patients may need multiple procedures to address various levels and structures. Last, in some patients obstructive sleep apnea may coincide with other disorders of sleep that can significantly affect their symptoms. Surgery should not be expected to improve excessive daytime sleepiness in patients where their apnea is "cured" but they continue to have significant sleep restriction or insomnia.

Focusing on improving airflow by reconstructing the soft tissues has led to the development of some newer techniques such as expansion sphincteroplasty, lateral pharyngoplasty, and palatal advancement. Some of these techniques are modifications of older procedures but with a new emphasis on modifying tissues to improve airflow. In some pediatric patients, more traditional procedures like adenotonsillectomy are sufficient although there are emerging data suggesting additional therapies may also be needed. Clinical outcomes assessing individual techniques in a multilevel disease where multiple interventions are used is difficult. Despite this, some reconstructive techniques of the soft tissues in the upper airway of patients with obstructive sleep apnea can be very beneficial.

REFERENCES

1. Powell NB, Guilleminault C. Rationale and indications for surgical treatment in obstructive sleep apnea. Otolaryngol Head Neck Surg 1991;2:87–90.
2. Riley RW, Powell NB, Li KK, et al. Surgery and obstructive sleep apnea: long-term clinical outcomes. Otolaryngol Head Neck Surg 2000; 122(3):415–21.
3. Dempsy JA, Skatrud JB, Jacques AJ, et al. Anatomical determinates of sleep disordered breathing across the spectrum of clinical and non-clinical subjects. Chest 2002;122:40–51.
4. Schwab RJ, Pierson R, Pasirstein M, et al. Family aggregation of upper airway soft tissue structures in normals and patients with sleep apnea. Am J Respir Crit Care Med 2006;173:453–63.
5. Hillman DR, Platt PR, Eastwood PR. The upper airway during anaesthesia. Br J Anaesth 2003; 91(1):31–9.
6. Mickelson SA, Hakim I. Is postoperative intensive care monitoring necessary after uvulopalatopharyngoplasty? Otolaryngol Head Neck Surg 1998; 119(4):352–6.
7. Friedman M, Ibrahim H, Bass L. Clinical staging for sleep-disordered breathing. Otolaryngol Head Neck Surg 2002;127(1):13–21.
8. Motta J, Guilleminault C, Schroeder JS, et al. Tracheostomy and hemodynamic changes in sleep-inducing apnea. Ann Intern Med 1978;89(4):454–8.
9. Friedman M, Tanyeri H, Lim JW, et al. Effect of improved nasal breathing on obstructive sleep apnea. Otolaryngol Head Neck Surg 2000;122(1):71–4.
10. Li HY, Lin Y, Chen NH, et al. Improvement in quality of life after nasal surgery alone for patients with obstructive sleep apnea and nasal obstruction. Arch Otolaryngol Head Neck Surg 2008;134(4):429–33.
11. Sugiura T, Noda A, Nakata S, et al. Influence of nasal resistance on initial acceptance of continuous positive airway pressure in treatment for obstructive sleep apnea syndrome. Respiration 2007;74(1): 56–60.
12. Buccheri A, Dilella G, Stella R. Rapid palatal expansion and pharyngeal space. Cephalometric evaluation. Prog Orthod 2004;5(2):160–71.
13. Compadretti GC, Tasca I, Bonetti GA. Nasal airway measurements in children treated by rapid maxillary expansion. Am J Rhinol 2006;20(4): 385–93.
14. Brietzke SE, Gallagher D. The effectiveness of tonsillectomy and adenoidectomy in the treatment of pediatric obstructive sleep apnea/hypopnea syndrome: a meta-analysis. Otolaryngol Head Neck Surg 2006;134(6):979–84.
15. Goldbart AD, Goldman JL, Veling MC, et al. Leukotriene modifier therapy for mild sleep-disordered breathing in children. Am J Respir Crit Care Med 2005;172(3):364–70.
16. Gozal D. Sleep-disordered breathing and school performance in children. Pediatrics 1998;102 (3 Pt 1):616–20.
17. Mitchell RB, Kelly J. Long-term changes in behavior after adenotonsillectomy for obstructive sleep apnea syndrome in children. Otolaryngol Head Neck Surg 2006;134(3):374–8.
18. Guilleminault C, Li K, Quo S, et al. A prospective study on the surgical outcomes of children with sleep-disordered breathing. Sleep 2004;27(1):95–100.

19. Mitchell RB, Kelly J. Behavior, neurocognition and quality-of-life in children with sleep-disordered breathing. Int J Pediatr Otorhinolaryngol 2006; 70(3):395–406.

20. Mitchell RB, Kelly J. Outcomes and quality of life following adenotonsillectomy for sleep-disordered breathing in children. ORL J Otorhinolaryngol Relat Spec 2007;69(6):345–8.

21. Guilleminault C, Quo S, Huynh NT, et al. Orthodontic expansion treatment and adenotonsillectomy in the treatment of obstructive sleep apnea in prepubertal children. Sleep 2008;31(7):953–7.

22. Li HY, Chen NH, Shu YH, et al. Changes in quality of life and respiratory disturbance after extended uvulopalatal flap surgery in patients with obstructive sleep apnea. Arch Otolaryngol Head Neck Surg 2004;130(2):195–200.

23. Cahali MB. Lateral pharyngoplasty: a new treatment for obstructive sleep apnea hypopnea syndrome. Laryngoscope 2003;113(11):1961–8.

24. Fujita S. Pharyngeal surgery for obstructive sleep apnea. In: Fairbanks D, DNFS, Ikematsu E, et al, editors. Snoring and obstructive sleep apnea. New York: Raven Press; 1987. p. 101–28.

25. Cahali MB, Formigoni GG, Gebrim EM, et al. Lateral pharyngoplasty versus uvulopalatopharyngoplasty: a clinical, polysomnographic and computed tomography measurement comparison. Sleep 2004;27(5): 942–50.

26. Pang KP, Woodson BT. Expansion sphincter pharyngoplasty: a new technique for the treatment of obstructive sleep apnea. Otolaryngol Head Neck Surg 2007;137(1):110–4.

27. Woodson BT, Robinson S, Lim HJ. Transpalatal advancement pharyngoplasty outcomes compared with uvulopalatopharygoplasty. Otolaryngol Head Neck Surg 2005;133(2):211–7.

28. Osman EZ, Abo-Khatwa MM, Hill PD, et al. Palatal surgery for snoring: objective long-term evaluation. Clin Otolaryngol Allied Sci 2003;28(3): 257–61.

29. Pang KP, Terris DJ. Snoring: simple to obstructive apnea. In: KH C, editor. Geriatric otolaryngology. New York: Taylor & Francis; 2006. p. 429–36.

30. Littner M, Kushida CA, Hartse K, et al. Practice parameters for the use of laser-assisted uvulopalatoplasty: an update for 2000. Sleep 2001;24(5): 603–19.

31. Ferguson KA, Heighway K, Ruby RR. A randomized trial of laser-assisted uvulopalatoplasty in the treatment of mild obstructive sleep apnea. Am J Respir Crit Care Med 2003;167(1):15–9.

32. Mair EA, Day RH. Cautery-assisted palatal stiffening operation. Otolaryngol Head Neck Surg 2000; 122(4):547–56.

33. Pang KP, Terris DJ. Modified cautery-assisted palatal stiffening operation: new method for treating snoring and mild obstructive sleep apnea. Otolaryngol Head Neck Surg 2007;136(5):823–6.

34. Stuck BA, Maurer JT, Hein G, et al. Radiofrequency surgery of the soft palate in the treatment of snoring: a review of the literature. Sleep 2004;27(3):551–5.

35. Brietzke SE, Mair EA. Injection snoreplasty: extended follow-up and new objective data. Otolaryngol Head Neck Surg 2003;128(5):605–15.

36. Maurer JT, Hein G, Verse T, et al. Long-term results of palatal implants for primary snoring. Otolaryngol Head Neck Surg 2005;133(4):573–8.

37. Nordgard S, Stene BK, Skjostad KW, et al. Palatal implants for the treatment of snoring: long-term results. Otolaryngol Head Neck Surg 2006;134(4):558–64.

38. Woodson BT. A tongue suspension suture for obstructive sleep apnea and snorers. Otolaryngol Head Neck Surg 2001;124(3):297–303.

39. DeRowe A, Gunther E, Fibbi A, et al. Tongue-base suspension with a soft tissue-to-bone anchor for obstructive sleep apnea: preliminary clinical results of a new minimally invasive technique. Otolaryngol Head Neck Surg 2000;122(1):100–3.

40. Kezirian EJ, Goldberg AN. Hypopharyngeal surgery in obstructive sleep apnea: an evidence-based medicine review. Arch Otolaryngol Head Neck Surg 2006;132(2):206–13.

41. Steward DL, Weaver EM, Woodson BT. Multilevel temperature-controlled radiofrequency for obstructive sleep apnea: extended follow-up. Otolaryngol Head Neck Surg 2005;132(4):630–5.

42. Vilaseca I, Morello A, Montserrat JM, et al. Usefulness of uvulopalatopharyngoplasty with genioglossus and hyoid advancement in the treatment of obstructive sleep apnea. Arch Otolaryngol Head Neck Surg 2002;128(4):435–40.

43. Woodson BT, Fujita S. Clinical experience with lingualplasty as part of the treatment of severe obstructive sleep apnea. Otolaryngol Head Neck Surg 1992;107(1):40–8.

44. Chabolle F, Wagner I, Blumen MB, et al. Tongue base reduction with hyoepiglottoplasty: a treatment for severe obstructive sleep apnea. Laryngoscope 1999;109(8):1273–80.

45. Woodson BT. Innovative technique for lingual tonsillectomy and midline posterior glossectomy for obstructive sleep apnea. Operative Techniques in Otolaryngology 2007;18:20–8.

46. Neruntarat C. Hyoid myotomy with suspension under local anesthesia for obstructive sleep apnea syndrome. Eur Arch Otorhinolaryngol 2003;260(5):286–90.

47. Neruntarat C. Genioglossus advancement and hyoid myotomy: short-term and long-term results. J Laryngol Otol 2003;117(6):482–6.

48. Golz A, Goldenberg D, Westerman ST, et al. Laser partial epiglottidectomy as a treatment for obstructive sleep apnea and laryngomalacia. Ann Otol Rhinol Laryngol 2000;109(12 Pt 1):1140–5.

Management of Obstructive Sleep Apnea by Maxillomandibular Advancement

Scott B. Boyd, DDS, PhD

KEYWORDS
- Obstructive sleep apnea
- Transverse distraction osteogenesis
- Maxillomandibular advancement

Obstructive sleep apnea (OSA) is a common primary sleep disorder that occurs in up to 9% of women and 24% of men ages 30 to 60.[1] OSA is a condition characterized by repetitive partial or complete upper airway collapse during sleep. The ensuing reduction in airflow leads to hypoxia and subsequent arousals from sleep, producing sleep deprivation. The effect that OSA has on general health and wellbeing has been well documented.[2,3] OSA is associated with hypertension,[4–6] cardiovascular disease,[7–10] metabolic syndrome,[11,12] stroke, and possible premature death.[13] There is a reduction in quality of life,[14,15] including diminished social function and an increased rate of motor vehicle accidents.[16] Deficits in neuropsychological functioning occur, including diminished vigilance, executive functioning, and motor coordination.[17]

Nasal continuous positive airway pressure (CPAP) is considered the first and most effective form of therapy to treat OSA in adults.[18] Significant improvements in objective and subjective sleepiness, quality of life, and cognitive function have been demonstrated following the use of CPAP.[18] Although CPAP has been shown to be highly effective, virtually eliminating OSA, long-term acceptance and adherence to therapy are relatively low. When CPAP adherence is defined as greater than 4 hours of nightly use, 46% to 83% of patients with OSA have been reported to be nonadherent

to treatment.[19] CPAP also requires lifetime nightly use.

Maxillomandibular advancement (MMA) is an orthognathic surgical procedure that has been used to manage OSA in individuals who are noncompliant with CPAP therapy.[20,21] MMA is a site-specific procedure, performed for the purpose of creating an enlarged posterior airway space at multiple anatomic levels, including the nasopharynx, oropharynx, and hypopharynx.[22] MMA involves surgical facial advancement by performance of concomitant maxillary and mandibular osteotomies (**Fig. 1**). MMA has been shown to significantly improve OSA, with reported short-term success rates ranging from 75% to 100%.[22–25] It is considered to be comparable in clinical effectiveness to CPAP.[26] Preliminary reports indicate that much of the short-term benefit of MMA may be maintained a long-term basis.[27,28]

Although some surgeons have approached MMA as a stand-alone procedure,[22,25] others have advocated a staged approach to surgery.[23] In the staged protocol, a patient diagnosed with OSA will first undergo phase 1 surgery, which includes uvulopalatopharyngoplasty (UPPP) and possibly other adjunctive procedures, such as genioglossal advancement. If phase 1 surgery is not effective, the patient would proceed to phase 2 surgery, consisting of MMA.

Vanderbilt School of Medicine, CCC 3322 MCN 2103, 1161 21st Avenue South, Nashville, TN 37232-2103, USA
E-mail address: scott.boyd@vanderbilt.edu

Oral Maxillofacial Surg Clin N Am 21 (2009) 447–457
doi:10.1016/j.coms.2009.09.001
1042-3699/09/$ – see front matter © 2009 Elsevier Inc. All rights reserved.

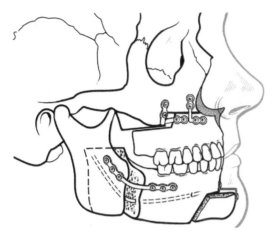

Fig. 1. Schematic diagram of maxillomandibular advancement procedure consisting of LeFort 1 maxillary osteotomy with step modification, bilateral sagittal split ramus osteotomies, and genial advancement. Shaded area depicts sites of piriform rim recontouring and anterior nasal spine reduction.

Overall the success rates for the staged protocol are high and yield reductions in sleep-disordered breathing and symptomology and high patient satisfaction.[23,28] The effectiveness of the individual stages of therapy, however, differs significantly. Although phase 2 surgery (MMA) has yielded success rates ranging from 93% to 100%,[23,28] the success rates for phase 1 surgery have varied between 22%[29] and 80%.[30] Overall, success rates for phase 1 are similar to those reported for isolated UPPP. Currently it is unknown whether staged surgery provides any benefit over isolated MMA. Recently, another form of staged surgery has been reported for treatment of patients with concomitant OSA and a maxillofacial skeletal deformity.[31,32] Distraction osteogenesis of the maxilla or mandible is performed as the first stage of therapy, followed by MMA as the second stage of treatment.

The main objective of this article is to provide practical guidelines for evaluating and managing OSA patients by MMA. The presentation will focus on MMA for adults, as this is the most common and clinically effective application of MMA to treat OSA.

PATIENT EVALUATION

The purpose of the initial surgical consultation is to confirm a diagnosis of OSA and to determine if the patient is a candidate for MMA. Commonly, the patient has been evaluated already by a sleep specialist and has undergone objective evaluation, by polysomnography, to establish a diagnosis of OSA. Furthermore, it is likely that the patient already has attempted to use CPAP. If this initial evaluation and treatment have occurred, the surgeon should confirm the findings; otherwise an overnight sleep study will need to be obtained to objectively establish a diagnosis of OSA before initiating any treatment. The patient also should be questioned about previous treatment of OSA and past response to therapy. This should include both the patient's subjective and objective (eg, post-treatment polysomnography [PSG]) response to therapy. Patients also should be questioned about any treatment-related adverse outcomes or complications of previous therapy.

The MMA surgical consultation visit combines the components of both a sleep evaluation for OSA and a routine orthognathic surgery consultation for correction of maxillofacial skeletal deformities (MSDs). Major components of the sleep evaluation include a comprehensive history, clinical examination, imaging studies, and sleep study. Although similar orthognathic surgical techniques are used to treat OSA, there are multiple important differences that exist between MSD and OSA patients. It is essential for the treating surgeon to understand these differences to facilitate effective and safe surgical care for the OSA patient. Important differences between the two groups include: goals of therapy, patient profile, underlying medical conditions, and magnitude of surgical movement. Most MSD patients are adolescents or young adults in good general health. In contrast, the typical OSA patient is a middle-aged, obese male, with significant comorbid medical conditions. The OSA patient has anatomic abnormalities of the upper airway, and larger surgical movements (10 mm or greater) of the maxilla and mandible routinely are required to effectively treat obstruction of the upper airway during sleep.

Symptoms and History

A thorough sleep-specific history and comprehensive medical history are essential components of the evaluation. Important elements of the sleep history include: presence and character of snoring, level of daytime sleepiness, self-reported or observed nocturnal episodes of breathing cessation, and the perceived quality and quantity of sleep. The Epworth Sleepiness Scale (ESS) is an eight-item questionnaire that commonly is used to subjectively assess the patient's level of daytime sleepiness.[33,34] The patient also may relate various symptoms related to a decreased quality of life, such as poor job performance, decreased ability to concentrate, memory loss, and fatigue. The Calgary Sleep Apnea Quality of Life Index (SAQLI)[35,36] and the Functional Outcomes of Sleep Questionnaire (FOSQ)[37] are two valid and reliable sleep-specific quality-of-life questionnaires that may be used.

A comprehensive medical history must be obtained, because OSA is associated with a wide spectrum of medical conditions that may affect surgical treatment and the patient's overall health. If there is presence or a suspicion of a significant medical condition, it will be important to obtain indicated consultations to establish the status of the disease, determine if the patient is a candidate for surgery, determine what can be done to optimize the patient's condition before surgery, and to obtain recommendations for intraoperative and postoperative management of the patient in regard to each significant medical condition. This assessment is essential to determine the risk/benefit ratio for surgical intervention. One of the most common medical conditions is hypertension, and it is important to optimize blood pressure preoperatively, because patients typically will have modified hypotensive anesthesia administered during surgery.

Physical Examination

A comprehensive head and neck examination should be performed for each patient. This physical examination should include measurement of the patient's body mass index (BMI), resting blood pressure, and neck circumference. The OSA clinical evaluation is very similar to a routine orthognathic surgery evaluation, with special attention directed to potential sites of upper airway obstruction.

It is important to carefully perform all aspects of the routine orthognathic surgery baseline clinical examination to facilitate surgical treatment planning and to determine if presurgical orthodontic care would be of benefit (**Fig. 2**). The clinical examination should include assessment of temporomandibular joint function and mandibular mobility, occlusion, status of the dentition, neurosensory function, and facial esthetics. For most middle-aged adults, adaptations in the dentition have occurred (eg, wear and restorations) to maximize occlusal relations of the teeth, and the patient may not benefit significantly from orthodontic therapy before surgery.

Important augmented components of the upper airway examination include: inspection of the nasal cavity to determine sites of possible obstruction and description of the size, character, and function of the tonsils, soft palate, lateral and posterior pharyngeal walls, and base of tongue. In addition to direct visual examination, endoscopic examination (fiberoptic nasopharyngoscopy) of the upper airway may be of benefit to aid in the visualization of the upper airway and identification of the site(s) of pharyngeal collapse and obstruction.

Imaging

A standardized lateral cephalometric radiograph should be taken, with the patient positioned in adjusted natural head position with the mandible in centric relation and the facial soft tissues in repose (see **Fig. 2**C). A cephalometric analysis then is performed to assist in the identification of potential sites of upper airway obstruction (posterior airway space) and to characterize craniofacial morphology. If the patient proceeds to surgery, the cephalometric radiograph will be used for both surgical treatment planning and assessment of changes in the facial skeleton and upper airway that occur as a result of surgery. The major limitation of the cephalometric radiograph is that obtaining the radiograph in an upright and awake position may not reflect the anatomic characteristics of the upper airway accurately when the patient is sleeping in a supine position.

Facial and intraoral digital photographs should be taken to document the clinical examination, and these may be linked to the lateral cephalometric radiograph to develop computerized surgical prediction images (see **Fig. 2**). This is important, because the magnitude of the surgical movement (10 mm or more of facial advancement) may have a significant impact on facial appearance. Additionally, the prediction images allow the patient to see the type (not necessarily the actual result) of facial esthetic changes that may occur as a result of surgery.

Computed tomography (CT) imaging has not been used routinely for the surgical treatment of adults with OSA. Because three-dimensional CT imaging recently has become available in an outpatient office setting (eg, cone beam technology), however, use of this technology may be beneficial. CT has the ability to visualize the entire upper airway and can demonstrate the association between three-dimensional changes in the facial skeleton as a result of surgery and the upper airway.

Indications for MMA

Once the evaluation has been completed, it can be determined if the patient is a surgical candidate. The indications for MMA are as follows:

Significant OSA (apnea + hypopnea index greater than 15) as objectively diagnosed by PSG, with concomitant symptoms

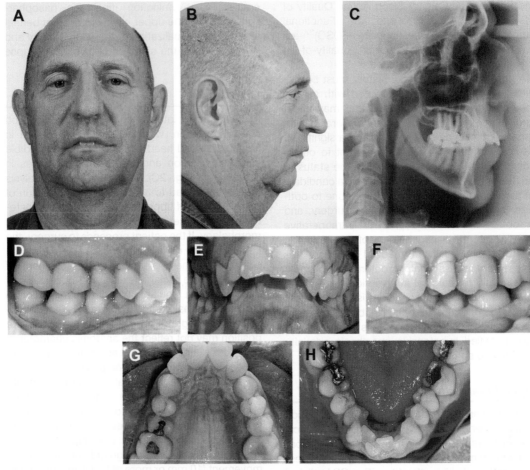

Fig. 2. Frontal facial (*A*), lateral facial (*B*), lateral cephalometric (*C*), and intraoral (*D–H*) pretreatment images of 59-year-old man with severe obstructive sleep apnea (AHI = 45), decreased posterior airway space, and concomitant maxillofacial skeletal deformities (mandibular retrognathia, transverse maxillary hypoplasia, and transverse mandibular hypoplasia). (*Modified from* Conley RS, Legan HL. Correction of severe obstructive sleep apnea with bimaxillary transverse distraction osteogenesis and maxillomandibular advancement. Am J Orthod Dentofacial Orthop 2006;129(2):284; with permission.)

Failure of CPAP because of nonacceptance or poor adherence to therapy

Craniofacial abnormalities (eg, children with micrognathia)

Ability to undergo surgical treatment (consideration of concomitant medical conditions)

It is also important to determine if the patient is a candidate for other forms of treatment. For example, if the patient has mild OSA, oral appliance therapy could be considered as a viable nonsurgical form of therapy. Bariatric surgery may be considered for the extremely obese patient (BMI greater than 35). Additionally, it should be determined if the patient is a candidate for surgical–orthodontic care, although this is uncommon.

Presurgical Treatment Planning

Because of the combined maxillary and mandibular movement and the large magnitude of facial advancement, it is recommended that a facebow transfer and mounting of dental casts on a semiadjustable articulator be used to provide an accurate assessment of the anatomic position of the maxilla and mandible. A model platform then is used to accurately simulate the planned three-dimensional movements of the maxilla and mandible. The final surgical plan will be based upon the patient's individual findings (eg, presence or absence of a pre-existing dentoskeletal deformity), but generally a minimum of 10 mm of mandibular advancement is recommended to produce the most improvement in OSA. In the patient who does not undergo concomitant orthodontic care, the maxilla will move an equivalent distance to the mandible, to maintain the patient's pre-existing occlusal relations.

Following completion of the model surgery, an interim splint is constructed using the advanced maxillary cast referenced to the uncut mounted mandibular cast (**Fig. 3**). The interim splint will facilitate accurate anteroposterior and transverse positioning of the maxilla, because the author's preferred sequence of surgery is to perform the maxillary surgery before the mandibular surgery. If the patient has an intact, stable dentition before surgery, it is unlikely that a final surgical splint will be necessary, because the patient can be placed in a stable, reproducible occlusion following performance of the maxillary and mandibular osteotomies.

SURGICAL TREATMENT
Anesthetic and Medical Management Considerations

It is very beneficial for the surgeon and attending anesthesiologist to discuss management of the airway, anesthetic techniques, and medical management of the patient before surgery to minimize the chance of perioperative complications. Fiberoptic nasopharyngeal intubation (possibly awake) with a Ring, Adair, Elwin tube provides a secure airway and ample access to the surgical field. A tracheotomy is not routinely indicated to secure the airway, but it is recommended where there is concern about the ability to safely perform nasopharyngeal intubation or where long-term postoperative airway management is required. Proper patient positioning and padding (eg, gel pads) are important to reduce the risk of pressure ischemia, which may be increased because of obesity, use of hypotensive anesthesia, and length of the procedure. Judicious intravenous fluid

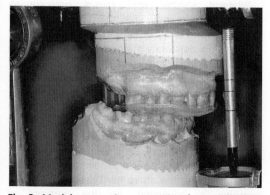

Fig. 3. Model surgery in preparation for maxillomandibular advancement showing 10 mm maxillary advancement and interim splint.

administration and use of intraoperative corticosteroids are helpful to diminish postoperative facial and parapharyngeal edema.

It is advantageous to use a modified hypotensive anesthetic technique during performance of the maxillary and mandibular osteotomies, to reduce blood loss and to improve visualization of the surgical field.[38] The ability to achieve this level of reduction in blood pressure depends upon the patient having a near-normal blood pressure preoperatively and underscores the importance of adequately treating any hypertension that was identified at the consultation visit. In addition to hypertension, patients with OSA may have a history of ischemic heart disease, myocardial infarction, and possibly stroke. In these individuals, it is especially important to maintain adequate organ perfusion. Although it is uncommon that blood transfusion will be necessary intraoperatively, the patient is presented the option of donating 2 units of autologous blood before surgery, so blood will be immediately available if needed.

Surgical Technique and Sequencing of Care

A LeFort 1 total maxillary osteotomy followed by bilateral sagittal split ramus osteotomies of the mandible are the author's preferred surgical technique and sequencing of care. Additionally, if indicated, a genial advancement is performed after completion of the maxillary and mandibular osteotomies. As a preliminary step, maxillary and mandibular arch bars are placed, unless the patient has undergone presurgical orthodontic care.

The LeFort 1 total maxillary osteotomy is performed using standard techniques[39] with a modified step design (**Fig. 4**).[40] The purpose of the step modification of the maxillary lateral wall osteotomies is to facilitate bony interfacing and presumably enhance the stability of the maxillary advancement. After completion of the osteotomy, the maxilla is mobilized until it can be passively positioned forward to the planned surgical position, as verified with the interim splint. To facilitate complete mobilization, slow, deliberate controlled force is used, usually in conjunction with a Rowe forceps (KLS-Martin, Jacksonville, FL). Force is modified accordingly to maintain adequate perfusion to the maxilla, which is monitored visually during the mobilization. The magnitude of the maxillary advancement may create a level of stimulation that produces a trigemino-cardiac reflex with resultant bradycardia or even asystole.[41] Release of stretch on the maxilla and associated soft tissues generally will stop the reflex and allow

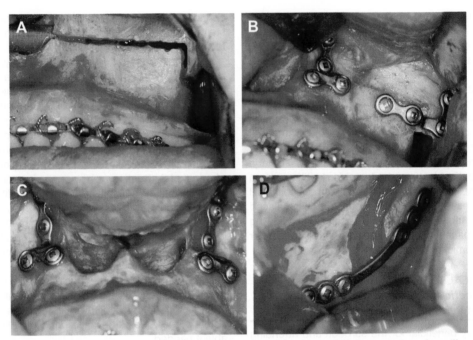

Fig. 4. Maxillomandibular advancement showing LeFort osteotomy with modified step design of maxillary lateral wall (*A*), placement of maxillary bone plates at piriform rim and zygomaticomaxillary buttress (*B*), piriform rim recontouring and reduction of anterior nasal spine (*C*), and placement of mono-cortical bone plate fixation of mandible, to minimize risk of injuring the inferior alveolar nerve (*D*).

the heart rate to return to normal. If the reflex inhibits the ability to adequately mobilize the maxilla, the reflex can be blocked by the use of atropine or glycopyrrolate. Adequate local anesthesia of the trigeminal nerve is also important to block the afferent pathway of the reflex.

Once the maxilla has been mobilized adequately, the interim splint is placed, and maxillomandibular fixation is secured. The complex then is passively rotated superiorly to the planned vertical position, as confirmed by an external reference pin. Judicious bone removal is performed as indicated, to remove any interference, in an effort to maximize bony interfacing. The piriform rim then is recontoured, and the anterior nasal spine is reduced (see **Fig. 1**) to minimize overprojection and widening of the nasolabial soft tissues that may occur as a result of the large advancement of the maxilla.

Then the maxilla is fixated with 2.0 mm L-shaped bone plates, placed at the piriform rim and zygomaticomaxillary buttress regions bilaterally, where the bone is thickest (see **Fig. 4**). The configuration of these plates produces a buttressing effect, which presumably enhances stability of the maxilla. Using this technique, the author has observed very good long-term stability of the maxilla and has not found it necessary to place any bone grafts. The potential benefits of not

having to perform a bone graft include: decreased operative time, elimination of any donor site morbidity, and earlier patient ambulation after surgery. Each of these factors is very important for a postoperative OSA patient who is obese and has medical comorbid conditions.

Once the patient is released from fixation and proper maxillary advancement has been confirmed, the maxillary soft tissue wound is closed using an alar base cinch suture and V-Y closure of the upper lip (at the midline). These two techniques are designed to maintain proper anatomic position of the nasolabial tissues.[42]

Bilateral sagittal split ramus osteotomies (BSSRO) of the mandible then are completed using standard techniques.[43] The mandible is split using a slow deliberate method of controlled force to facilitate visualization of the inferior alveolar nerve and diminish the chance of injury to the nerve. Minimizing surgical trauma to the inferior alveolar nerve is especially important, because OSA patients are generally middle-aged and presumably have a decreased ability to recover from a nerve injury.[44,45] Once the split is completed, care is taken to maintain soft tissue attachments so the entire hard tissue-soft tissue complex is advanced, for the purpose of increasing the posterior airway space. The mandibular osteotomies then are stabilized in the advanced position by either bone plates and monocortical screws, or three bicortical screws (see **Fig. 4**). After final assessment of maxillary and mandibular position, the mandibular wound is closed in standard fashion.

A genial advancement is performed if indicated, after completion of the LeFort 1 osteotomy and BSSRO. Various methods have been used for genial advancement, ranging from a standard genioplasty to a more isolated genial tubercle advancement. The main objective of the procedure is to advance the genioglossal musculature for the purpose of advancing the tongue and presumably increasing the posterior airway space.

Postoperative Care and Monitoring

Once the surgical procedure has been completed and the patient is sufficiently awake to meet criteria for extubation, the nasopharyngeal tube typically is removed in the operating room. This protocol has the advantage of having both the treating anesthesiologist and surgeon present at the time of extubation, as well as all necessary equipment immediately available if reintubation is necessary. Using this protocol, it is very uncommon for a patient to require reintubation. After extubation and stabilization, the patient is transported to the ICU for overnight monitoring. The patient's airway and associated medical conditions will need to be monitored closely. The patient is observed closely for any apneic events and oxygen supplementation is administered by face mask to maintain adequate oxygen saturation. Using this protocol, generally few apneic episodes, are observed and adequate oxygen saturations can be maintained, so postoperative CPAP has not been used routinely. For the first postoperative night, pain is controlled through the use of incremental intravenous dosing of narcotic analgesics. Close observation of the airway occurs during administration of the analgesics, as respiratory depression may occur at even low doses of narcotics in OSA patients.

Typically, the patient will be stable enough to be transferred to a step-down unit on the first postoperative day. Pain control can be maintained by a patient-controlled anesthesia (PCA) pump or liquid medications administered orally. Normal postoperative recovery will be initiated including ambulation and consumption of a liquid diet, similar to a typical orthognathic surgery patient.

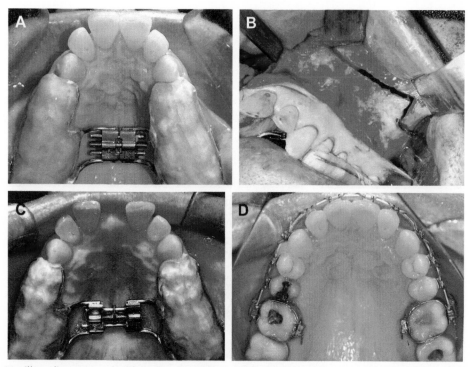

Fig. 5. Maxillary distraction of patient shown in **Fig. 2**. (*A*) Bonded maxillary expansion appliance. (*B*) Maxillary LeFort 1 osteotomy without downfracture and osteotome used for midpalatal osteotomy. (*C*) Completed transverse distraction of maxilla. (*D*) Pre-MMA alignment of maxillary dentition. (*Modified from* Conley RS, Legan HL. Correction of severe obstructive sleep apnea with bimaxillary transverse distraction osteogenesis and maxillomandibular advancement. Am J Orthod Dentofacial Orthop 2006;129(2):286; with permission.)

It is recommended that nighttime oxygen saturations be monitored by pulse oximetry until the patient can maintain near-normal oxygen saturations on room air while sleeping.

The typical hospital stay is 2 to 3 days. The patient then will be evaluated on an outpatient basis every 1 to 2 weeks for about 6 to 8 weeks following surgery. A nocturnal polysomnography study should be completed about 3 to 6 months following surgery to objectively evaluate treatment outcome.

Variations in Surgical Technique

Most of the OSA patients presenting for surgical treatment by MMA can be managed by the protocol that has been described. Some patients, however, will have OSA and a concomitant MSD. When present, the patient is a candidate for combined management of the MSD and OSA. Most maxillofacial skeletal deformities that occur in the vertical and anteroposterior dimensions can be treated by presurgical orthodontics followed by MMA. There will be a differential movement of the maxilla and mandible to facilitate correction of the MSD and the OSA. In development of the surgical plan, it is important to confirm that the mandibular advancement will be at least 10 mm, to ensure clinically effective treatment of OSA.

If a component of the MSD occurs in the transverse dimension, the patient may benefit from two-stage surgical treatment.[31] The first stage of treatment will include maxillary distraction osteogenesis (**Fig. 5**) and possibly mandibular symphyseal distraction osteogenesis (**Fig. 6**). The maxillary procedure is similar to a standard LeFort 1 maxillary osteotomy with a step design, without downfracture. The lateral wall step is modified slightly (by widening the bone cut), to facilitate transverse expansion without contacting the adjacent bone. If interferences exist, an open bite could be created during the distraction, as the posterior maxilla may ramp downward during the expansion. A midpalatal osteotomy then is completed to the posterior aspect of the hard palate, using an osteotome and mallet with digital palatal palpation to minimize the chance of perforating the mucosa. Once the osteotomy is completed, the appliance is activated temporarily about 1 to 2 mm to ensure that the maxilla can be expanded without significant resistance and the expansion is occurring without any boney interference. The inferior border and body of the

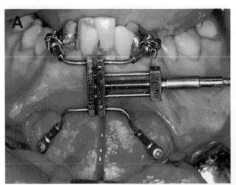
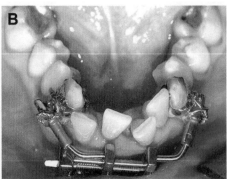
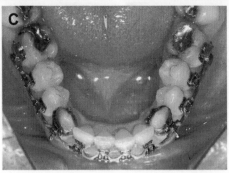

Fig. 6. Mandibular distraction of patient shown in **Fig. 2**. (*A*) Completed midline vertical symphyseal osteotomy with placement of combined tooth-borne and bone-borne distraction appliance. (*B*) Mandibular distraction in progress. (*C*) Pre-MMA alignment of mandibular dentition. (*Modified from* Conley RS, Legan HL. Correction of severe obstructive sleep apnea with bimaxillary transverse distraction osteogenesis and maxillomandibular advancement. Am J Orthod Dentofacial Orthop 2006;129(2):287; with permission.)

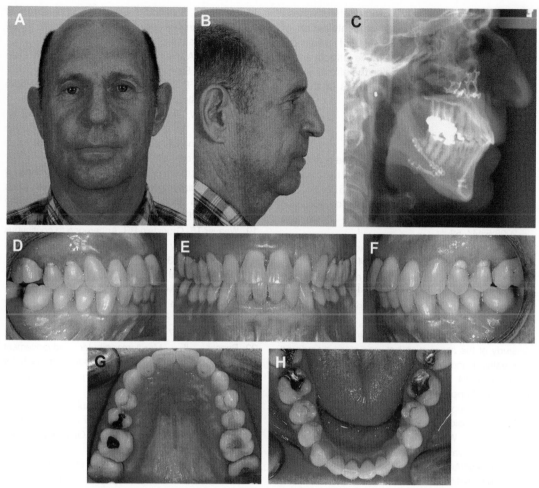

Fig. 7. Frontal facial (*A*), lateral facial (*B*), lateral cephalometric (*C*), and intraoral (*D–H*) post-treatment images of patient shown in **Fig. 2**, with successful treatment of severe obstructive sleep apnea (post-MMA AHI = 5), increased posterior airway space, and correction of maxillofacial skeletal deformities and malocclusion. (*Modified from* Conley RS, Legan HL. Correction of severe obstructive sleep apnea with bimaxillary transverse distraction osteogenesis and maxillomandibular advancement. Am J Orthod Dentofacial Orthop 2006;129(2):289; with permission.)

mandibular symphyseal osteotomy are completed with a reciprocating saw. A fine bur then is used to initiate the alveolar component of the osteotomy, and it then is completed using a fine spatula osteotome and mallet. Then the distraction osteogenesis appliance is secured to the mandible (see **Fig. 6**A). There is a latency period of 7 days before distraction is begun for the maxillary and mandibular osteotomies; this period is followed by distraction of 1 mm per day. Once the distraction is complete and the osseous segments have consolidated, conventional orthodontic therapy is performed to obtain well-coordinated and well-aligned dental arches (see **Fig. 5**D and **Fig. 6**C).[31] After completion of orthodontic therapy, MMA will be performed to treat both the OSA and remaining MSD (**Fig. 7**).

SUMMARY AND FUTURE DIRECTIONS

MMA is a clinically effective treatment alternative for individuals with obstructive sleep apnea, who cannot adhere to CPAP therapy. To date, published reports indicate that MMA is a very effective surgical treatment, especially for patients with severe OSA. Additionally, MMA, in conjunction with orthodontics and other reconstructive procedures (such as distraction osteogenesis), can be used to treat concomitant OSA and maxillofacial skeletal deformities. Accurate and comprehensive documentation of OSA treatment outcomes (both objective and subjective) has gained increased importance, as those responsible for paying for health care focus on the delivery of cost-effective care.[46] Treatment outcome research is needed to elucidate the long-term clinical effectiveness and safety of MMA, as well as identification of positive and negative predictors of treatment outcome. Additionally comparative effectiveness research is needed, to determine the effectiveness of MMA compared with other modes of therapy such as CPAP and oral appliances.

REFERENCES

1. Young T, Palta M, Dempsey J, et al. The occurrence of sleep-disordered breathing among middle-aged adults. N Engl J Med 1993;328:1230–5.

2. Eckert DJ, Malhotra A. Pathophysiology of adult obstructive sleep apnea. Proc Am Thorac Soc 2008;5:144–53.

3. Punjabi NR. The epidemiology of adult sleep apnea. Proc Am Thorac Soc 2008;5:136–43.

4. Nieto FJ, Young TB, Lind BK, et al. Association of sleep-disordered breathing, sleep apnea, and hypertension in a large community-based study. JAMA 2000;283:1829–36.

5. Peppard PE, Young T, Palta M, et al. Prospective study of the association between sleep-disordered breathing and hypertension. N Engl J Med 2000; 342:1378–84.

6. Young T, Peppard P, Palta M, et al. Population-based study of sleep-disordered breathing as a risk factor for hypertension. Arch Intern Med 1997;157:1745–52.

7. Somers VK, White DP, Amin R, et al. Sleep apnea and cardiovascular disease: an American Heart Association/American College of Cardiology Foundation Scientific Statement from the American Heart Association Council for High Blood Pressure Research Professional Education Committee, Council on Clinical Cardiology, Stroke Council, and Council on Cardiovascular Nursing. J Am Coll Cardiol 2008;52:686–717.

8. McNicholas WT, Bonsignore MR. Sleep apnoea as an independent risk factor for cardiovascular disease: current evidence, basic mechanisms and research priorities. Eur Respir J 2007;29:156–78.

9. Phillips B. Sleep-disordered breathing and cardiovascular disease. Sleep Med Rev 2005;9:131–40.

10. Shahar E, Whitney CW, Redline S, et al. Sleep-disordered breathing and cardiovascular disease. Cross sectional results of the sleep heart health study. Am J Respir Crit Care Med 2001;163:19–25.

11. Vgontzas AN, Bixler EO, Chrousos GP. Sleep apnea is a manifestation of the metabolic syndrome. Sleep Med Rev 2005;9:211–24.

12. Lam JCM, Ip MSM. An update on obstructive sleep apnea and the metabolic syndrome. Curr Opin Pulm Med 2007;13:484–9.

13. He J, Kryger MH, Zorich FJ, et al. Mortality and apnea index in obstructive sleep apnea. Experience in 385 male patients. Chest 1988;94:9–14.

14. Moyer CA, Sonnad SS, Garetz SL, et al. Quality of life in obstructive sleep apnea: a systematic review of the literature. Sleep Med 2001;2:477–91.

15. Reimer MA, Flemons WW. Quality of life in sleep disorders. Sleep Med Rev 2003;7:335–49.

16. George CFP, Smiley A. Sleep apnea and automobile crashes. Sleep 1999;22:790–5.

17. Beebe DW, Groesz L, Wells C, et al. The neuropsychological effects of obstructive sleep apnea: a meta-analysis of norm-referenced and case-controlled data. Sleep 2003;26(3):298–307.

18. Giles TL, Lasserson TJ, Smith BH, et al. Continuous positive airways pressure for obstructive sleep apnoea in adults. Cochrane Database Syst Rev 2006;(3):CD001106.

19. Weaver TE, Grunstein RR. Adherence to continuous positive airway pressure therapy. Proc Am Thorac Soc 2008;5:173–8.

20. Li KK. Surgical therapy for adult obstructive sleep apnea. Sleep Med Rev 2005;9:201–9.

21. Pirsig W, Verse T. Long-term results in the treatment of obstructive sleep apnea. Eur Arch Otorhinolaryngol 2000;257:570–7.

22. Prinsell JR. Maxillomandibular advancement surgery in a site-specific treatment approach for obstructive sleep apnea in 50 consecutive patients. Chest 1999;116:1519–29.

23. Riley RW, Powell NB, Guilleminault C. Obstructive sleep apnea syndrome: a review of 306 consecutively treated surgical patients. Otolaryngol Head Neck Surg 1993;108:117–25.

24. Waite PD, Wooten V, Lachner J, et al. Maxillomandibular advancement surgery in 23 patients with obstructive sleep apnea syndrome. J Oral Maxillofac Surg 1989;47:1256–61.

25. Hochban W, Brandenburg U, Peter JH. Surgical treatment of obstructive sleep apnea by maxillomandibular advancement. Sleep 1994;17(7): 624–9.

26. Epstein LJ, Kristo D, Strollo PJ, et al. Clinical guideline for the evaluation, management, and long-term care of obstructive sleep apnea in adults. J Clin Sleep Med 2009;5(3):263–76.

27. Conradt R, Hochban W, Brandenburg U, et al. Long-term follow-up after surgical treatment of obstructive sleep apnea by maxillomandibular advancement. Eur Respir J 1997;10:123–8.

28. Riley RW, Powell NB, Li KK, et al. Surgery and obstructive sleep apnea: long-term clinical outcomes. Otolaryngol Head Neck Surg 2000;122:415–21.

29. Bettega G, Pepin J, Veale D, et al. Obstructive sleep apnea syndrome. Fifty-one consecutive patients treated by maxillofacial surgery. Am J Respir Crit Care Med 2000;162:641–9.

30. Dattilo DJ, Drooger SA. Outcome assessment of patients undergoing maxillofacial procedures for the treatment of sleep apnea: comparison of

subjective and objective results. J Oral Maxillofac Surg 2004;62(2):164–8.

31. Conley RS, Legan HL. Correction of severe obstructive sleep apnea with bimaxillary transverse distraction osteogenesis and maxillomandibular advancement. Am J Orthod Dentofacial Orthop 2006;129(2):283–92.

32. Guilleminault C, Li KK. Maxillomandibular expansion for the treatment of sleep-disordered breathing: preliminary result. Laryngoscope 2004;114(5): 893–6.

33. Johns MW. A new method for measuring daytime sleepiness: the epworth sleepiness scale. Sleep 1991;14:50–5.

34. Johns MW. Reliability and factor analysis of the epworth sleepiness scale. Sleep 1992;15:376–81.

35. Flemons WW, Reimer MA. Development of a disease-specific health-related quality-of-life questionnaire for sleep apnea. Am J Respir Crit Care Med 1998;158:494–503.

36. Flemons WW, Reimer MA. Measurement properties of the Calgary sleep apnea quality-of-life index. Am J Respir Crit Care Med 2002;159:159–64.

37. Weaver TE, Laizner AM, Evans LK, et al. An instrument to measure functional status outcomes for disorders of excessive sleepiness. Sleep 1997;20: 835–43.

38. Choi WS, Samman N. Risks and benefits of deliberate hypotension in anaesthesia: a systematic review. Int J Oral Maxillofac Surg 2008;37: 687–703.

39. Bell WH. Le Fort I osteotomy for correction of maxillary deformities. J Oral Surg 1975;44:412–26.

40. Kaminishi RM, Davis WH, Hochwald DA, et al. Improved maxillary stability with modified LeFort I technique. J Oral Maxillofac Surg 1983;41: 203–5.

41. Lang S, Lanigan DT, van der Wal M. Trigeminocardiac reflexes: maxillary and mandibular variants of the oculocardiac reflex. Can J Anaesth 1991;38(6): 757–60.

42. Conley RS, Boyd SB. Facial soft tissue changes following maxillomandibular advancement for treatment of obstructive sleep apnea. J Oral Maxillofac Surg 2007;65(7):1332–40.

43. Epker BN. Modifications in the sagittal osteotomy of the mandible. J Oral Surg 1977;35:157–62.

44. Bays RA, Bouloux GF. Complications of orthognathic surgery. Oral Maxillofacial Surg Clin N Am 2003;15: 229–42.

45. MacIntosh RB. Experience with the sagittal osteotomy of the mandibular ramus: a 13-year review. J Oral Maxillofac Surg 1981;8:151.

46. Weaver TE. Outcome measurement in sleep medicine practice and research. Part I: assessment of symptoms, subjective and objective daytime sleepiness, health-related quality of life and functional status. Sleep Med Rev 2001;5:103–28.

Management of Obstructive Sleep Apnea: Role of Distraction Osteogenesis

Carl Bouchard, DMD, MSc, FRCD (C)*, Maria J. Troulis, DDS, MSc, Leonard B. Kaban, DMD, MD

KEYWORDS

- Distraction osteogenesis • Obstructive sleep apnea
- Orthognathic surgery • Maxillomandibular advancement
- Respiratory disturbance index

In the past, oral and maxillofacial surgeons were consulted on patients with obstructive sleep apnea (OSA) only when other methods of treatment, such as continuous positive airway pressure, dental appliances, and soft tissue operations, failed.[1–6] Maxillomandibular advancement (MMA) to enlarge the skeleton and thereby expand the soft tissue airway was a treatment of "last resort." With time, the high level of success achieved by MMA has been well documented[5–10] and oral and maxillofacial surgeons are now regularly consulted by sleep medicine physicians and OSA patients earlier in the course of disease.

The indications for distraction osteogenesis (DO) in patients with OSA include infants and children with airway obstruction as a result of congenital micrognathia or midface hypoplasia (**Fig. 1**). These patients may have Treacher Collins or Nager syndromes, craniofacial microsomia, syndromic or nonsyndromic Robin sequence, and syndromic or nonsyndromic midface hypoplasia. They have OSA as a result of severe micrognathia, short posterior face height, malposition of the tongue base,[11] or midface deficiency and choanal atresia. A significant number of these patients are tracheostomy-dependent and they require large advancements (>15 mm) to adequately improve the upper airway. Because of the magnitude of advancement needed, DO is the treatment of choice. The ultimate goal is to prevent tracheostomy or to decannulate the trachea in patients who already have a surgical airway.

OSA may also occur in adults with mandibular or maxillary retrognathia manifest by a convex profile and a short chin-to-throat distance (**Fig. 2**). Occasionally, these patients may have an orthognathic profile. The magnitude of advancement required to successfully manage OSA (10–15 mm) in these adults is less than in patients with congenital or infant airway obstruction. The advancement can often be achieved by standard osteotomies and acute lengthening. DO is chosen if the patient is unwilling to accept the risk of inferior alveolar nerve paresthesia with standard orthognathic surgery or if special circumstances (eg, multiple operations for cleft lip/palate, large magnitudes of advancement, maxillofacial radiation therapy) prevent successful skeletal expansion by traditional osteotomies.

This article discusses the role of DO in the management of airway obstruction and OSA.

This project was funded in part by the AO Foundation (Berne, Switzerland); Synthes CMF (West Chester, PA); MGH Department of OMFS Education & Research Fund; and the Hanson Foundation (Boston, MA).
Department of Oral and Maxillofacial Surgery, Massachusetts General Hospital, Harvard School of Dental Medicine, Boston, MA 02114, USA
* Corresponding author.
E-mail address: carlbouch@hotmail.com (C. Bouchard).

oralmaxsurgery.theclinics.com

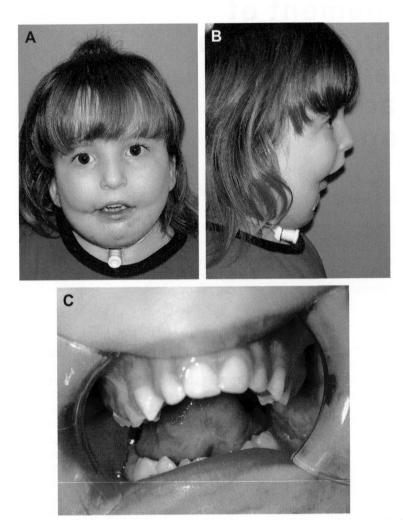

Fig. 1. Frontal (*A*), lateral (*B*), and intraoral (*C*) preoperative photographs of a 2-year-old girl with first and second pharyngeal arch deformity. The resultant micrognathia has necessitated a long-term tracheostomy to secure her upper airway.

PREOPERATIVE EVALUATION
History and Physical Examination

The diagnosis of OSA is established on the basis of history, physical examination, polysomnography, and the appropriate radiologic evaluation. History and physical examination in adults with OSA is similar, whether standard orthognathic surgery or DO is contemplated. When considering DO in patients with congenital or infant airway obstruction, specific elements in the history and physical examination should be evaluated.

Signs and symptoms of children with OSA vary with age.[12] These children may present with retarded growth, poor eating, crying spells, daytime fatigue, enuresis, poorly established day-night sleeping cycles, and so forth.[12–14] Parents may not associate these symptoms with abnormal sleeping or airway obstruction.[12]

The physical examination should include a thorough nasal and oropharyngeal evaluation. This is especially true because lymphoid tissue hypertrophy is a frequent cause of snoring and airway obstruction in infants and toddlers.[15] In these cases, soft tissue procedures, such as tonsillectomy and adenoidectomy, may be curative.[15] The craniofacial skeleton should be evaluated to identify anomalies that predispose to airway obstruction, such as maxillary or mandibular hypoplasia. The presence of excessive overjet, crossbite, and the morphology of the palate and tongue must be noted. The physical evaluation is often completed with fiberoptic nasopharyngoscopy.[16]

Radiographic Evaluation

Traditionally, lateral cephalograms have been used to evaluate the airway anatomy of patients

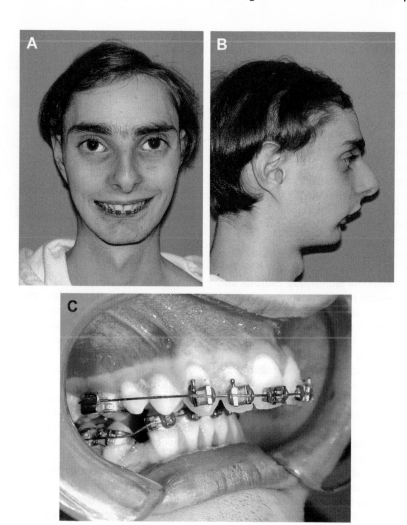

Fig. 2. Frontal (*A*), lateral (*B*), and intraoral (*C*) preoperative photographs of a 17-year-old patient with a nonsyndromic severe mandibular retrognathia.

with OSA. The advantages of plain radiographs include low radiation dose, low cost, widespread availability, familiarity, and high comfort level for most surgeons. Commonly used lateral cephalometric measurements are posterior airway space and hyoid to mandibular plane distance, although no association between these measurements and airway obstruction has been definitively established.[17] Lateral cephalograms and panoramic radiographs are also useful for assessing progression of distraction, vector of distraction, and formation of the regenerate before removal of the distraction devices. Ultrasound has also been documented as a noninvasive, radiation-free, low-cost alternative to plain radiographs and CT to evaluate the regenerate after DO.[18]

CT scans provide accurate three-dimensional images of the upper airway and allow calculation of volumes, cross-sectional areas, and parameters of shape. There have been numerous reports documenting abnormalities of size and shape of the upper airway in OSA patients using three-dimensional CT data.[19–23] At Massachusetts General Hospital, three-dimensional CT scans are routinely used to evaluate these upper airway parameters in patients with OSA. Three-dimensional CT data are also critical for planning skeletal expansion by DO to calculate vectors of movement, to localize osteotomies, to properly orient distraction devices, and to localize screw holes for distractor footplates.[24–26]

DISTRACTION OSTEOGENESIS
General Comments

DO is a technique of bone lengthening that uses the body's healing potential to form new bone. An osteotomy is created and a distraction device is rigidly fixed to the bone. After a latency period of 0 to 7 days to allow upregulation of bone metabolism, the device is activated at a rate of 1 mm/day. Tension across the osteotomy induces bone formation and histiogenesis of blood vessels, muscles, nerves, cartilage, ligaments, skin and mucosa.[27–29]

DO was first reported in 1905 by Codivilla[30] and popularized in the 1950s by Ilizarov, a Russian orthopedic surgeon.[31] The first report of mandibular DO for human patients was in 1992 by McCarthy and colleagues.[32] Mandibular lengthening by DO is now a frequently used technique to correct congenital and acquired craniofacial deformities requiring skeletal expansion.[24,25]

DO is a minimally invasive alternative to standard osteotomies and acute bone lengthening. The operation is of lesser magnitude and shorter duration than traditional techniques. Skeletal and soft tissue expansion of great magnitude can be achieved without the use of bone grafts and soft tissue flaps.[32] Overall morbidity is reduced and, at least theoretically, relapse rate is diminished because gradual bone lengthening results in soft tissue hyperplasia and hypertrophy rather than stretching. DO can also be used in patients with compromised soft tissue (eg, multiply operated cleft patients or those who have had radiation therapy).

DO requires precise preoperative planning to ensure that the correct vector of distraction is executed. Patients undergoing this operation must be carefully selected to ensure that they, or their families, are able to adequately activate and care for the appliances. In addition, the overall treatment time is longer and more postoperative visits are required for patients who undergo DO versus those who have standard osteotomies. This is to monitor wound care, oral hygiene, proper appliance activation, vector of movement, and formation of the regenerate.[26]

Preoperative Planning

Photographs, face-bow articulated dental models, three-dimensional CT, panoramic and cephalometric radiographs are obtained for diagnosis and treatment planning. The proper vector of distraction is established using the lateral cephalogram or three-dimensional CT.

For unidirectional mandibular elongation in the sagittal plane an occlusal surgical navigation device is fabricated. The device consists of an acrylic occlusal splint indexed to the teeth with posterior metallic extensions that are used intraoperatively to guide bone cuts (**Fig. 3**). The guide is positioned on the teeth and the osteotomy marked parallel to the metal rod extension. After

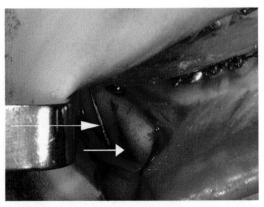

Fig. 3. An acrylic occlusal splint with metallic extensions (*long arrow*) is used to mark the osteotomy (*short arrow*).

completion of corticotomies, the distractor footplates are secured across the osteotomy with screws. In most cases, the vector of distraction is established at 110 degrees to the mandibular occlusal plane.

For more complex anatomy and skeletal movements, three-dimensional treatment planning is mandatory, particularly if a buried distraction device is used. Unlike extraoral pin-retained devices, buried distractors do not allow midcourse corrections of the vector of distraction. Planning must be accurate.[26] Three-dimensional CT data are imported into a treatment planning software program (Osteoplan, Harvard Surgical Planning Lab, Brigham and Women's Hospital, Boston, Massachusetts) developed in collaboration with the Harvard Surgical Planning Laboratory.[33] Reproducible landmarks are identified and the osteotomies located.[33–35] With the cutting tool, the planned osteotomies are virtually performed and the bone segments moved to the anticipated final position (**Fig. 4**).

The system identifies potential areas of bony interferences between the displaced segment of bone and adjacent structures along the path of movement. If such interferences are encountered, the vector of distraction should be modified or the interferences eliminated at the time of distractor placement. For example, a coronoidectomy may have to be performed to prevent collision between the coronoid process and the skull base in patients with hemifacial microsomia undergoing ramus lengthening by DO (**Fig. 5**). If a curvilinear distractor is to be used, the software calculates the proposed axis of movement on each side, the radii of curvature of the devices, and their lengths and orientation.[36]

Correct placement and orientation of the osteotomies and distraction devices are critical for the success of the treatment. To accurately transfer

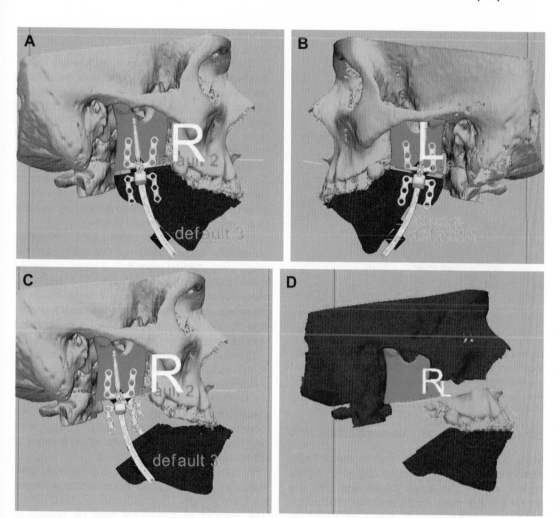

Fig. 4. Preoperative three-dimensional CT scan images are imported into the treatment planning software (Osteoplan). (*A*) The proposed osteotomy on the right (*From* Kaban LB, Seldin E, Everett P, et al. Clinical application of curvilinear distraction osteogenesis for correction of mandibular deformities. J Oral Maxillofac Surg 2009;67:996–1008; with permission) and (*B*) on the left are virtually executed and distractor devices are oriented (proximal segment in green, distal segment in blue). (*C*) The software then executes the predetermined movement. The accuracy of the vector is verified and anatomic interferences identified. (*From* Kaban LB, Seldin E, Everett P, et al. Clinical application of curvilinear distraction osteogenesis for correction of mandibular deformities. J Oral Maxillofac Surg 2009;67:996–1008; with permission.) (*D*) The final position of the jaws after mandibular distraction and a LeFort I osteotomy is illustrated (maxilla in light green).

the virtual plan from the software, a three-dimensional stereolithographic model of the skull is created from the CT scan. The osteotomies are made on the model and acrylic stents are constructed to fit the area to be distracted. The osteotomies are marked on the stents and these are used to transfer the osteotomy, distractor, and footplate locations to the patient intraoperatively (**Fig. 6**).[37]

For midface advancement by DO, surgical planning depends on the type of distractor used. Rigid external distraction (RED) devices are easily installed and the vector can be modified, if necessary, during the activation period.[38] For these reasons, three-dimensional treatment planning with stereolithographic models and surgical guides may not be necessary. Currently available internal midface distractors are unidirectional and the vector cannot be changed once the device is fixed in place. The complex anatomy of the maxilla makes accurate intraoperative distractor placement difficult. Three-dimensional treatment planning and the use of a stereolithographic model on which to prebend and orient the distractors are necessary for correct orientation of the osteotomies and to secure the appliances in the ideal position (**Fig. 7**).[39,40]

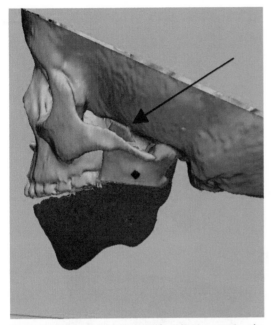

Fig. 5. In this case of left hemifacial microsomia, the treatment planning software (Osteoplan) anticipated a collision between the coronoid process and the skull base (*arrow*). To complete the distraction without interferences, a coronoidectomy was performed.

CONGENITAL AND INFANT AIRWAY OBSTRUCTION

Many children with congenital craniomaxillofacial anomalies have at least some degree of airway obstruction. In the acute phase and with the proper training, many cases of airway obstruction can be managed by parents using special feeding, positioning, and suctioning techniques.[41] Some patients require a tracheostomy during the neonatal period, however, to prevent the morbidity and mortality of acute and long-term airway obstruction.[42] Bypassing the upper airway is an extremely effective treatment for OSA, but tracheostomy is associated with complications and morbidity and requires significant home care responsibilities on the part of the parents and caregivers.[43] Tracheomalacia, chronic bronchitis, laryngeal stenosis, delayed speech acquisition, and compromised psychosocial interactions are among the numerous complications reported.[43–46] Because obstruction is often in the retroglossal area, advancing the mandible displaces the tongue base forward and prevents collapse of the oropharynx during sleep. The large advancements required to successfully treat syndromic and nonsyndromic congenital micrognathia are difficult to achieve with standard osteotomies and the relapse rate is unacceptably high (**Fig. 8**).[11] Skeletal expansion by DO in this group of patients seems to be more stable and less morbid than standard osteotomies with or without bone grafting.[47,48]

The timing of DO in children with severe micrognathia to prevent tracheostomy or to achieve decannulation is controversial. Steinbacher and colleagues[11] suggest that DO should be delayed until the child is at least 2 years of age. The authors point out that in infants, bone stock is limited and the tooth buds restrict options for placement and fixation of the distractor and compromise stability. Furthermore, during the first 2 years of life, natural growth of the mandible and increase in neuromuscular tone may be sufficient to obviate the need for distraction in nonsyndromic children.

Steinbacher and colleagues[11] reported successful decannulation of five tracheostomy-dependent children older than 2 years of age. All these patients were syndromic and tracheostomy-dependent beginning in infancy. Because there was no resolution of airway obstruction by age 2, the permanent decannulation achieved was attributed to the mandibular lengthening.

Burstein and Williams[49] also reported satisfactory results in infants and children with Robin syndrome treated by DO. In a series of 20 patients, 14 avoided tracheostomy and 5 were permanently decannulated. Monasterio and colleagues[50] reported improvement in swallowing, sleep apnea, and hypopnea after mandibular DO in a series of 18 patients with Robin syndrome.

In patients with syndromic and nonsyndromic midface hypoplasia, advancements of large magnitude are required to improve airway obstruction. The amount of movement may be difficult to achieve and may be limited by the soft tissue resistance. The potential for relapse is greater after standard, one-stage midface advancement versus gradual lengthening by DO.[14,51,52] This is especially true in patients with cleft lip and palate.[53–55] DO also eliminates the need for bone grafting and its potential donor site morbidity. Improvement in airway obstruction has been demonstrated in patients with midfacial distraction.[14,56–59] Midface advancement increases the dimension of the airway at the level of the nasopharynx.

Increased nasal resistance early in life has been shown to affect the development of the upper jaw.[60–63] Nasal septal deviation or turbinate hypertrophy reduces airflow through the nose and this affects the transverse dimension of the palate.[64] Maxillary expansion (ME) by DO increases the intranasal space and improves nasal airflow.[64–67] Indirect improvement is also observed by a modification of the resting position of the tongue.[68] Pirelli and colleagues[64] have demonstrated the efficacy of ME for the treatment of OSA in 31 children who did not have adenoid hypertrophy or obesity.

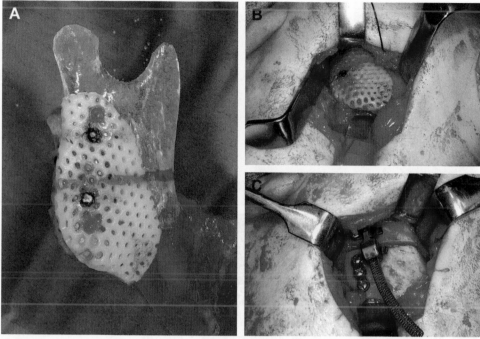

Fig. 6. Surgical stents were fabricated on a stereolithographic model for this case of bilateral mandibular curvilinear distraction. (*A*) The right stent demonstrates the planned osteotomy (red line) and the screw holes for the footplates of the device. (*B*) Intraoperative photographs demonstrating the stent in place. (*C*) The completed osteotomy and distractor placement. (*From* Kaban LB, Seldin E, Everett P, et al. Clinical application of curvilinear distraction osteogenesis for correction of mandibular deformities. J Oral Maxillofac Surg 2009;67:996–1008; with permission.)

All the patients included in this study had a normal apnea hypopnea index 4 months postoperatively. Guilleminault and colleagues[69] studied the impact of tonsillectomy and adenoidectomy and ME on OSA in prepubertal children. Half of the patients (N = 32) had ME followed by tonsillectomy and adenoidectomy and the other half had the same treatment but in reverse order. All patients required both operations to be cured, except two patients who were completely cured after ME alone.

Surgical Procedure

Unidirectional mandibular advancement by DO

The operation is performed under general anesthesia with nasoendotracheal intubation or by way of a pre-existing tracheostomy. The mandible is exposed by an intraoral incision and corticotomies are performed with the aid of a navigation device. An appropriate semiburied distraction device (eg, Leibinger, Dallas, Texas; or Synthes CMF, West Chester, Pennsylvania) with detachable footplates is fixed across the osteotomy with 2-mm screws (**Fig. 9**). The appliance is activated to ensure proper function and to verify that

the osteotomy is complete. Distraction is initiated 48 to 96 hours after the operation at a rate of 1 mm/day. The rhythm of distraction varies from twice to four times a day, depending on patient comfort. Radiographs are obtained immediately postoperatively, to confirm correct distractor placement.

Patients are evaluated every week during the activation phase and every other week during the consolidation period. Bone healing is evaluated by clinical and radiologic examination. End-DO radiographs document the final jaw position (**Fig. 10**). The regenerate can also be evaluated by sequential ultrasonography, limiting the amount of radiation to the patients.[70]

Three-dimensional, curvilinear mandibular DO

Children with severe micrognathia usually require multivector distraction because of the combination of a short mandibular body, short ramus and condyle unit, and steep mandibular plane. Currently available multivector distractors are large and cumbersome to accommodate the multiple joints necessary to distract in three dimensions. They also require close monitoring and multiple adjustments during the activation

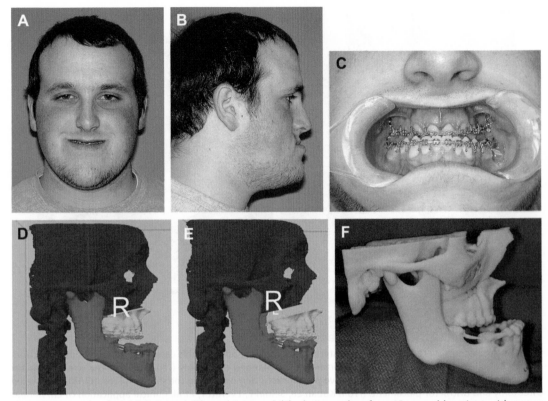

Fig. 7. Preoperative facial (*A*), lateral (*B*), and intraoral (*C*) photographs of an 18-year-old patient with severe maxillary sagittal hypoplasia. Because of the large advancement required, it was decided move the maxilla forward gradually by distraction osteogenesis with internal devices. (*D*) The proposed osteotomy was executed with the surgical planning software (Osteoplan) and (*E*) the anticipated final position of the maxilla determined. (*F*) A stereolithographic model was created to prebend the devices and facilitate their placement.

phase to minimize the risk of a poor occlusal and esthetic result.

Seldin and colleagues described the concept of three-dimensional curvilinear distraction and demonstrated the use of a semiburied fixed-trajectory curvilinear distractor in a mini pig model.[26] They subsequently reported the use of curvilinear distraction in a series of 13 patients.[37] The device is less complicated for the patient than an external multivector device and the three-dimensional movement accomplished by curvilinear distraction can correct most mandibular deformities. Most importantly, it can advance the mandible in the sagittal plane, rotate it in a counterclockwise direction, and lengthen the ramus-condyle unit.

Miller and colleagues reported successful management of 12 infants with micrognathia and obstructive sleep apnea by curvilinear distraction osteogenesis.[71,72,73] All 12 infants had successful mandibular lengthening and the obstructive component improved with minimal complications. The improvement was documented by pre- and

postoperative polysomnograms in 6 of the patients.

A virtual model is created from the three-dimensional CT scan using Osteoplan (see **Fig. 4**). The osteotomy is performed on the virtual model and the desired vector of movement in each plane is calculated by the software. A prescription for the distractor with the required radius of curvature is created.[33,35]

Depending on the ramus size and the specific anatomy, an intraoral or a submandibular approach is used to expose the mandible. Stents are used to correctly execute the osteotomy and position the distractors (see **Fig. 6**). The device is activated until a wedge-shaped gap is demonstrated and then the distractor is turned back to the neutral position. The usual distraction protocol is respected with regard to latency period, activation rhythm, and consolidation time.

Midfacial DO

Patients with syndromic and nonsyndromic midfacial hypoplasia and airway obstruction can be

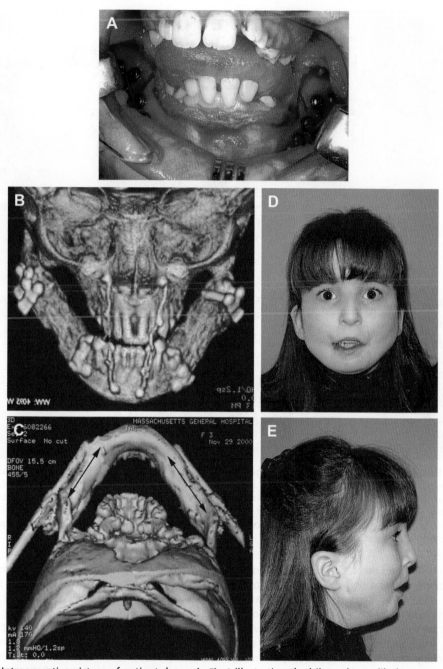

Fig. 8. (*A*) Intraoperative picture of patient shown in **Fig. 1** illustrating the bilateral mandibular osteotomies and the internal distractor placement. (*B, C*) End distraction three-dimensional CT scan demonstrating the regenerate (*arrows*). Postoperative frontal (*D*) and lateral (*E*) pictures. The patient was permanently decannulated.

treated by midfacial DO using a RED device or a semiburied device (**Fig. 11**). The midface can be advanced at the LeFort I, LeFort II, or Le Fort III level depending on the anatomic deformity and the patient's age. After completion of the appropriate osteotomy, the selected distractor is fixed in place. The RED consists of an orthodontic dental splint attached to the upper teeth with external traction hooks that are contoured around the upper lip and bent up to the level of the palatal plane. The splint can be cemented in place or secured to the upper teeth with circumdental wires. The device can also be anchored to the bone with extraoral traction wires. The external hooks are then connected to a halo that is screwed to the cranium.

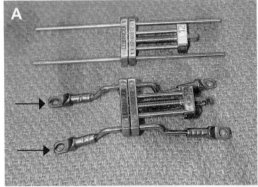
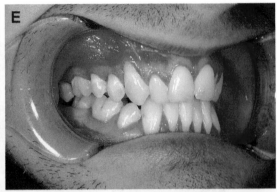
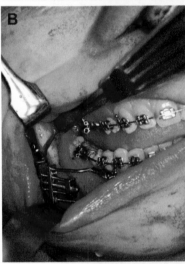
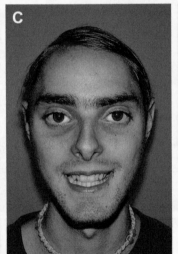
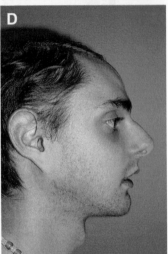

Fig. 9. (*A*) Semi-buried distraction device (Leibinger, Dallas, Texas) is used for unidirectional mandibular advancement. The device (*top*) is bent to conform to the patient's anatomy (*bottom*). The proximal footplates are notched (*arrows*) for easy removal. (*B*) The appliance is installed by an intraoral incision and it is secured across the osteotomy with two screws on the proximal segment, one on the distal segment, and the remaining footplate is attached to the adjacent tooth with a circumdental wire. Postoperative frontal (*C*), lateral (*D*), and intraoral (*E*) photographs of patient shown in **Fig. 2**.

Internal distractors are secured on each side of the osteotomy by adapting the footplates to the proximal and distal segments of the maxilla. Extension pins can be attached to the distractors to assess the vector and parallelism of the devices (**Fig. 12**). Prior adaptation of the distractors on a stereolithographic model facilitates placement and ensures a correct vector of distraction.

LATER-ONSET OSA

In nonsyndromic adult patients, the facial anomalies may be more subtle. These patients present with mandibular retrognathia, bi-maxillary retrusion, or even an orthognathic profile. They are typically older (>40 years) and overweight (body mass index >30). Numerous reports have demonstrated the efficacy of MMA for the treatment of OSA.[6–8] This can be achieved with traditional orthognathic

surgery with the expectation of a stable result in most patients. These patients, however, who often have significant comorbidities, are at risk for significant complications. This has led some surgeons to seek minimally invasive alternatives to achieve MMA. Adult patients over age 40 concerned with the risk for inferior alveolar nerve injury and patients with compromised soft tissue (eg, scarring from previous surgeries or radiation therapy) are candidates for MMA by DO.

Paoli and colleagues[74] reported the use of mandibular DO, followed by a LeFort I osteotomy for the treatment of OSA. By staging the procedure, they were able to distract the mandible until normalization of polysomnography data, respiratory disturbance index, or apnea hypopnea index. The distractor was removed at the time of the second operation, and the maxilla was advanced to recreate the preoperative occlusion. In contrast

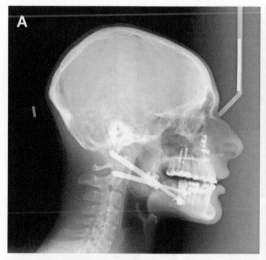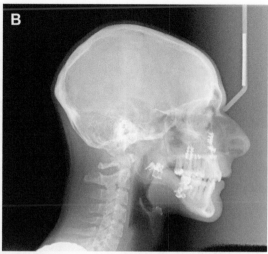

Fig. 10. (*A*) End of distraction lateral cephalometric radiograph of patient shown in **Fig. 2**. Posterior airway space was significantly increased. (*B*) After the consolidation period, the devices are removed, but the footplates are left in place.

to bimaxillary distraction, this protocol does not require the use of intermaxillary fixation and converts one major surgical intervention into two less invasive operations. The major inconvenience is the temporary malocclusion created during the distraction and the consolidation phase, which can last up to 3 months. Also, the patient is submitted to the risk of two general anesthetics.

In a case series of five patients treated with mandibular DO (N = 4) and bi-maxillary DO (N = 1), Li and colleagues[75] obtained an improvement of the respiratory disturbance index from a mean preoperative 49.3 events per hour to 6.6 events per hour postoperatively. The mean distraction distance was 8.1 mm (5.5–12.5 mm). No major complications were reported and only temporary paresthesia of the inferior alveolar nerve was observed. The authors pointed out the importance of establishing the correct vector of distraction, particularly in this group of patients that usually refuse to undergo an orthodontic treatment. If a malocclusion is created, orthodontic compensation is not possible.

Magliocca and Helman[76] reported the use of a bimaxillary distractor (KLS Martin, Jacksonville, Florida) that is attached on the maxilla and on the mandible simultaneously. Once they obtained the desired advancement, a polysomnography was performed. If the patient did not meet their criteria for the cure of OSA, distraction was continued. They obtained a 100% cure rate with this technique on nine male patients.

Wang and colleagues[77] published the largest series of patients treated by DO for OSA. They studied the impact of mandibular advancement

on OSA on 28 patients with micrognathia. Twenty-three patients were completely cured and five had mild OSA at the end of the treatment. However, most patients in this study had micrognathia secondary to unilateral or bilateral temporomandibular joint ankylosis, and no maxillary distraction was performed.

DISCUSSION

Successful treatment of OSA can be achieved by a variety of medical and surgical modalities. The high success rate of MMA has been established and oral and maxillofacial surgeons are now involved more frequently and at an earlier stage in the treatment of OSA.[6–10] Because of the magnitude, morbidity, and potential instability of standard surgical techniques for large expansions of the facial skeleton, the use of DO as a minimally invasive alternative has become commonplace.[11,77–79]

DO is an alternative for acute bone lengthening in situations requiring large movements not attainable by standard osteotomies, acute lengthening, and bone grafting. Advancements of 20 mm or more without a bone graft and the associated donor site morbidity, scarring, and potential for infection can be achieved. Soft tissue seems to grow linearly along lines of tension, and skin, muscles, nerves, and vascular tissue are generated, not stretched.[80] Resistance to advancement by the soft tissue envelope is decreased by this process of distraction histogenesis.[81] The advantage is obvious, especially for severe midface hypoplasia and micrognathia where the stretched soft tissue

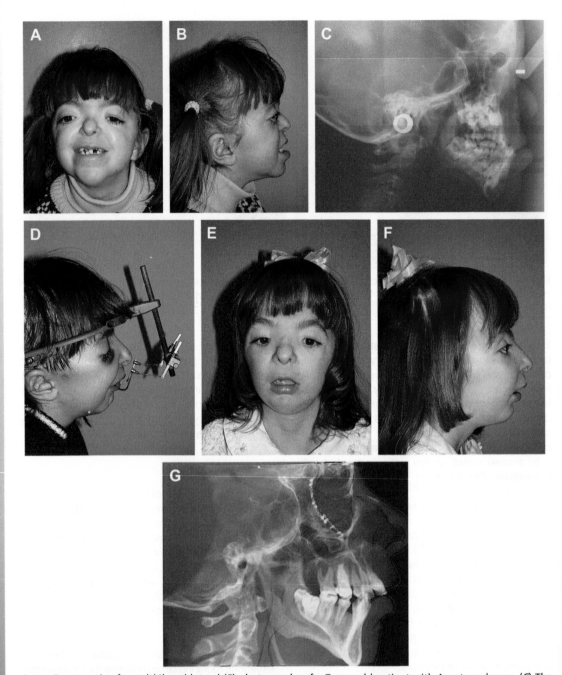

Fig. 11. Preoperative frontal (*A*) and lateral (*B*) photographs of a 7-year-old patient with Apert syndrome. (*C*) The lateral cephalometric radiograph demonstrates the severe midface retrusion and the constriction of the upper airway at the retropalatal area. (*D*) Patient underwent a midface advancement with a rigid external distractor attached to the upper teeth. Postoperative frontal (*E*) and lateral (*F*) photographs. (*G*) The postoperative lateral cephalometric radiograph demonstrates an increase in the retropalatal area. (*Courtesy of* Bonnie L. Padwa, DMD, MD, Boston, MA.)

envelope contributes to relapse after traditional osteotomies, acute lengthening, and bone grafts. Scarring from previous operations (cleft lip and palate repair, uvulopalatopharyngoplasty, orthognathic surgery) or radiation therapy may limit the amount of advancement possible by standard orthognathic surgical procedures. These patients are ideal candidates for DO.

In animal studies, it has been reported that there are no histologic alterations in nerve fibers after

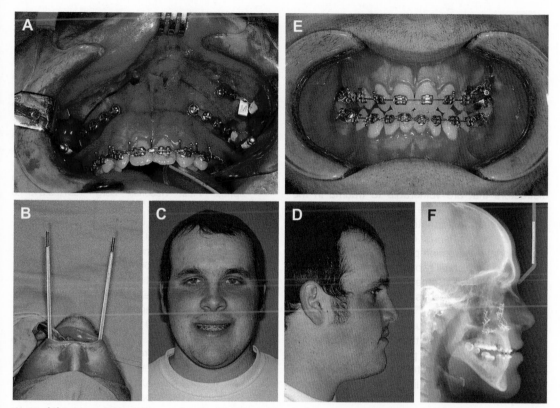

Fig. 12. (*A*) Intraoperative picture of patient in **Fig. 7**. The devices are secured across the osteotomy gap. (*B*) The vector of distraction is verified with extension pins and should be parallel to each other. Postoperative frontal (*C*), lateral (*D*), and intraoral (*E*) photographs. (*F*) Postoperative lateral cephalometric radiograph.

small and large mandibular advancements by DO.[82,83] The few clinical studies published on the incidence of inferior alveolar nerve injury after DO demonstrate favorable neurosensory outcomes when compared with bilateral sagittal split osteotomies in patients over 40 years of age.[47,84,85] DO is an excellent alternative for older patients concerned about the risk of inferior alveolar nerve injury with bilateral sagittal split osteotomy.

Patients and families should be informed that the overall length of treatment and the number of postoperative visits are significantly increased after DO when compared with standard osteotomies.[86] Because patients play an important role in the execution of DO, there is a greater requirement for patient understanding and cooperation.[87] Failure to follow the prescribed activation can result in inappropriate vector of distraction, inadequate regenerate formation and even dismantling of the distractor. With bimaxillary DO, a prolonged period of maxillomandibular fixation is necessary, affecting speech, alimentation, and social interaction. During the process of distraction, patients may experience pain, problems sleeping, and disturbances of recreational activities.[88]

Distraction devices have become smaller and less cumbersome.[24,25] Buried, miniature devices are better tolerated by patients, but because midcourse corrections are not possible, they require more precise and sophisticated treatment planning to ensure the correct vector of distraction.

Advantages of external distractors include relatively easy placement, avoidance of complex plate bending, ability to modify the vector of distraction during the activation phase, and ability to remove the appliance in the office without the need for a second operation or general anesthesia.[89] However, external devices are inconvenient and cumbersome and may be uncomfortable.

Incorrect vector of distraction is a common complication of DO. Mofib and colleagues[90] reported the incidence of an incorrect vector during unidirectional distraction in 3278 patients to be as high as 8.8%. Accurate preoperative planning using three-dimensional CT scans and construction of intraoperative surgical navigation aids should markedly diminish this complication.

An incomplete osteotomy may result in extreme pain, bending or dismantling of the distractor, and inadequate skeletal expansion. This problem can be detected clinically and radiographically by noting a discrepancy between the number of activations and the bony gap created. Ultimately, if unrecognized, this results in premature healing of the osteotomy. Incomplete osteotomy can be avoided by activating the device intraoperatively to confirm separation of the bone segments.

During the activation phase, mechanical problems, such as screw loosening, hardware fracture, and dislodgment of the device can complicate the treatment. This is particularly true with external distractors that are vulnerable to trauma in the younger child. Premature consolidation or inadequate regenerate formation, in the absence of distractor problems, is often the result of an inappropriate distraction protocol.[91]

The long-term stability of DO has not been definitively established. Some authors have demonstrated stable results,[48,92–97] and others a tendency for relapse.[98–100] These studies are difficult to compare because of the different protocols used to evaluate the results. Inadequate duration of consolidation, poor preoperative orthodontic preparation, posturing, and myoskeletal anomalies have all been linked to poor long-term stability.[101,102]

SUMMARY

DO to expand the facial skeleton is an alternative to standard orthognathic surgery for selected patients with OSA. For children with congenital micrognathia or midface hypoplasia, DO allows large advancements without the need for bone grafting and with less risk of relapse. For later-onset OSA, DO may represent an alternative when acute bone movement is expected to be difficult (scarring from previous surgery or radiation therapy) or when the risk for inferior alveolar nerve damage is unacceptable (patients older than 40 years).

REFERENCES

1. Reeves-Hoche MK, Meck R, Zwillich CW, et al. An objective evaluation of patient compliance. Am J Respir Crit Care Med 1994;149:149–54.
2. Waldhorn RE, Herrick TW, Nguyen MC, et al. Long-term compliance with nasal continuous positive airway pressure therapy of obstructive sleep apnea. Chest 1990;97:33–8.
3. Sher AE, Schechtman KB, Piccirillo JF. The efficacy of surgical modifications of the upper airway in adults with obstructive sleep apnea syndrome. Sleep 1996;19:156–77.
4. Li KK, Powell NB, Riley RW, et al. Overview of phase I surgery for obstructive sleep apnea syndrome. Ear Nose Throat J 1999;78:836–7, 841–45.
5. Li KK, Riley RW, Powell NB, et al. Overview of phase II surgery for obstructive sleep apnea syndrome. Ear Nose Throat J 1999;78:851, 854–7.
6. Riley RW, Powell NB, Guilleminault C. Obstructive sleep apnea syndrome: a review of 306 consecutively treated surgical patients. Otolaryngol Head Neck Surg 1993;108:117–25.
7. Hochban W, Conradt R, Brandenburg U, et al. Surgical maxillofacial treatment of obstructive sleep apnea. Plast Reconstr Surg 1997;99:619–26 [discussion: 27-8].
8. Waite PD, Wooten V, Lachner J, et al. Maxillomandibular advancement surgery in 23 patients with obstructive sleep apnea syndrome. J Oral Maxillofac Surg 1989;47:1256–61 [discussion: 62].
9. Prinsell JR. Maxillomandibular advancement surgery in a site-specific treatment approach for obstructive sleep apnea in 50 consecutive patients. Chest 1999;116:1519–29.
10. Bettega G, Pepin JL, Veale D, et al. Obstructive sleep apnea syndrome: fifty-one consecutive patients treated by maxillofacial surgery. Am J Respir Crit Care Med 2000;162:641–9.
11. Steinbacher DM, Kaban LB, Troulis MJ. Mandibular advancement by distraction osteogenesis for tracheostomy-dependent children with severe micrognathia. J Oral Maxillofac Surg 2005;63:1072–9.
12. Guilleminault C, Lee JH, Chan A. Pediatric obstructive sleep apnea syndrome. Arch Pediatr Adolesc Med 2005;159:775–85.
13. Lauritzen C, Lilja J, Jarlstedt J. Airway obstruction and sleep apnea in children with craniofacial anomalies. Plast Reconstr Surg 1986;77:1–6.
14. Nelson TE, Mulliken JB, Padwa BL. Effect of midfacial distraction on the obstructed airway in patients with syndromic bilateral coronal synostosis. J Oral Maxillofac Surg 2008;66:2318–21.
15. Postic WP, Shah UK. Nonsurgical and surgical management of infants and children with obstructive sleep apnea syndrome. Otolaryngol Clin North Am 1998;31:969–77.
16. Goldberg AN, Schwab RJ. Identifying the patient with sleep apnea: upper airway assessment and physical examination. Otolaryngol Clin North Am 1998;31:919–30.
17. Miles PG, Vig PS, Weyant RJ, et al. Craniofacial structure and obstructive sleep apnea syndrome: a qualitative analysis and meta-analysis of the literature. Am J Orthod Dentofacial Orthop 1996;109:163–72.
18. Thurmuller P, Troulis M, O'Neill MJ, et al. Use of ultrasound to assess healing of a mandibular distraction wound. J Oral Maxillofac Surg 2002;60:1038–44.

19. Lan Z, Itoi A, Takashima M, et al. Difference of pharyngeal morphology and mechanical property between OSAHS patients and normal subjects. Auris Nasus Larynx 2006;33:433–9.

20. Vos W, De Backer J, Devolder A, et al. Correlation between severity of sleep apnea and upper airway morphology based on advanced anatomical and functional imaging. J Biomech 2007;40:2207–13.

21. Li HY, Chen NH, Wang CR, et al. Use of 3-dimensional computed tomography scan to evaluate upper airway patency for patients undergoing sleep-disordered breathing surgery. Otolaryngol Head Neck Surg 2003;129:336–42.

22. Verin E, Tardif C, Buffet X, et al. Comparison between anatomy and resistance of upper airway in normal subjects, snorers and OSAS patients. Respir Physiol 2002;129:335–43.

23. Caballero P, Alvarez-Sala R, Garcia-Rio F, et al. CT in the evaluation of the upper airway in healthy subjects and in patients with obstructive sleep apnea syndrome. Chest 1998;113:111–6.

24. McCarthy JG, Staffenberg DA, Wood RJ, et al. Introduction of an intraoral bone-lengthening device. Plast Reconstr Surg 1995;96:978–81.

25. Diner PA, Kollar EM, Martinez H, et al. Intraoral distraction for mandibular lengthening: a technical innovation. J Craniomaxillofac Surg 1996;24:92–5.

26. Seldin E, Troulis M, Kaban LB. Evaluation of a semi-buried fixed-trajectory curvilinear distraction device in an animal model. J Oral Maxillofac Surg 1999;57:1442–6.

27. Aronson J, Good B, Stewart C, et al. Preliminary studies of mineralization during distraction osteogenesis. Clin Orthop Relat Res 1990;43–9.

28. Aronson J, Harrison B, Boyd CM, et al. Mechanical induction of osteogenesis: preliminary studies. Ann Clin Lab Sci 1988;18:195–203.

29. Aronson J, Harrison BH, Stewart CL, et al. The histology of distraction osteogenesis using different external fixators. Clin Orthop Relat Res 1989;241:106–16.

30. Codivilla A. On the means of lengthening, in the lower limbs, the muscle and tissues which are shortened through deformity. Am J Orthop Surg 1904;2:353–69.

31. Ilizarov GA. The principles of the Ilizarov method. Bull Hosp Jt Dis Orthop Inst 1988;48:1–11.

32. McCarthy JG, Schreiber J, Karp N, et al. Lengthening the human mandible by gradual distraction. Plast Reconstr Surg 1992;89:1–8 [discussion: 9–10].

33. Troulis MJ, Everett P, Seldin EB, et al. Development of a three-dimensional treatment planning system based on computed tomographic data. Int J Oral Maxillofac Surg 2002;31:349–57.

34. Yeshwant K, Seldin EB, Gateno J, et al. Analysis of skeletal movements in mandibular distraction osteogenesis. J Oral Maxillofac Surg 2005;63:335–40.

35. Yeshwant KC, Seldin EB, Kikinis R, et al. A computer-assisted approach to planning multidimensional distraction osteogenesis. Atlas Oral Maxillofac Surg Clin North Am 2005;13:1–12.

36. Ritter L, Yeshwant K, Seldin EB, et al. Range of curvilinear distraction devices required for treatment of mandibular deformities. J Oral Maxillofac Surg 2006;64:259–64.

37. Kaban LB, Seldin E, Everett P, et al. Clinical application of curvilinear distraction osteogenesis for correction of mandibular deformities. J Oral Maxillofac Surg 2009;67:996–1008.

38. Kahn DM, Schendel SA. Distraction osteogenesis of the maxilla at the LeFort I level using internal distractor. In: Bell WH, Guerrero CA, editors. Distraction osteogenesis of the facial skeleton. Hamilton: BC Decker; 2007. p. 267–71.

39. Gateno J, Engel ER, Teichgraeber JF, et al. A new Le Fort I internal distraction device in the treatment of severe maxillary hypoplasia. J Oral Maxillofac Surg 2005;63:148–54.

40. Kessler P, Wiltfang J, Schultze-Mosgau S, et al. Distraction osteogenesis of the maxilla and midface using a subcutaneous device: report of four cases. Br J Oral Maxillofac Surg 2001;39:13–21.

41. Schaefer RB, Stadler III JA, Gosain AK. To distract or not to distract: an algorithm for airway management in isolated Pierre Robin sequence. Plast Reconstr Surg 2004;113:1113–25.

42. Levine OR, Simpser M. Alveolar hypoventilation and cor pulmonale associated with chronic airway obstruction in infants with down syndrome. Clin Pediatr (Phila) 1982;21:25–9.

43. Guilleminault C, Simmons FB, Motta J, et al. Obstructive sleep apnea syndrome and tracheostomy: long-term follow-up experience. Arch Intern Med 1981;141:985–8.

44. Zeitouni A, Manoukian J. Tracheotomy in the first year of life. J Otolaryngol 1993;22:431–4.

45. Arola MK. Tracheostomy and its complications: a retrospective study of 794 tracheostomized patients. Ann Chir Gynaecol 1981;70:96–106.

46. Puhakka HJ, Kero P, Valli P, et al. Tracheostomy in pediatric patients. Acta Paediatr 1992;81:231–4.

47. Whitesides LM, Meyer RA. Effect of distraction osteogenesis on the severely hypoplastic mandible and inferior alveolar nerve function. J Oral Maxillofac Surg 2004;62:292–7.

48. Swennen G, Schliephake H, Dempf R, et al. Craniofacial distraction osteogenesis: a review of the literature: Part 1: clinical studies. Int J Oral Maxillofac Surg 2001;30:89–103.

49. Burstein FD, Williams JK. Mandibular distraction osteogenesis in Pierre Robin sequence:

application of a new internal single-stage resorbable device. Plast Reconstr Surg 2005;115:61–7 [discussion: 8–9].

50. Monasterio FO, Molina F, Berlanga F, et al. Swallowing disorders in Pierre Robin sequence: its correction by distraction. J Craniofac Surg 2004;15: 934–41.

51. Fearon JA. The LeFort III osteotomy: to distract or not to distract? Plast Reconstr Surg 2001;107: 1091–103.

52. Mixter RC, David DJ, Perloff WH, et al. Obstructive sleep apnea in Apert's and Pfeiffer's syndromes: more than a craniofacial abnormality. Plast Reconstr Surg 1990;86:457–63.

53. Posnick JC, Dagys AP. Skeletal stability and relapse patterns after Le Fort I maxillary osteotomy fixed with miniplates: the unilateral cleft lip and palate deformity. Plast Reconstr Surg 1994;94: 924–32.

54. Hochban W, Ganss C, Austermann KH. Long-term results after maxillary advancement in patients with clefts. Cleft Palate Craniofac J 1993;30: 237–43.

55. Cheung LK, Samman N, Hui E, et al. The 3-dimensional stability of maxillary osteotomies in cleft palate patients with residual alveolar clefts. Br J Oral Maxillofac Surg 1994;32:6–12.

56. Fearon JA. Halo distraction of the Le Fort III in syndromic craniosynostosis: a long-term assessment. Plast Reconstr Surg 2005;115:1524–36.

57. Cedars MG, Linck II DL, Chin M, et al. Advancement of the midface using distraction techniques. Plast Reconstr Surg 1999;103:429–41.

58. Mathijssen I, Arnaud E, Marchac D, et al. Respiratory outcome of mid-face advancement with distraction: a comparison between Le Fort III and frontofacial monobloc. J Craniofac Surg 2006;17:880–2.

59. Meling TR, Hans-Erik H, Per S, et al. Le Fort III distraction osteogenesis in syndromal craniosynostosis. J Craniofac Surg 2006;17:28–39.

60. Vargervik K, Miller AJ, Chierici G, et al. Morphologic response to changes in neuromuscular patterns experimentally induced by altered modes of respiration. Am J Orthod 1984;85:115–24.

61. Linder-Aronson S. Dimensions of face and palate in nose breathers and habitual mouth breathers. Odontologisk Revy 1969;14:187–200.

62. Harvold EP, Tomer BS, Vargervik K, et al. Primate experiments on oral respiration. Am J Orthod 1981;79:359–72.

63. Miller AJ, Vargervik K, Chierici G. Sequential neuromuscular changes in rhesus monkeys during the initial adaptation to oral respiration. Am J Orthod 1982;81:99–107.

64. Pirelli P, Saponara M, Guilleminault C. Rapid maxillary expansion in children with obstructive sleep apnea syndrome. Sleep 2004;27:761–6.

65. Timms DJ. Rapid maxillary expansion in the treatment of nocturnal enuresis. Angle Orthod 1990; 60:229–33 [discussion: 34].

66. Timms DJ. The effect of rapid maxillary expansion on nasal airway resistance. Br J Orthod 1986;13: 221–8.

67. Timms DJ. The reduction of nasal airway resistance by rapid maxillary expansion and its effect on respiratory disease. J Laryngol Otol 1984;98: 357–62.

68. Principato JJ. Upper airway obstruction and craniofacial morphology. Otolaryngol Head Neck Surg 1991;104:881–90.

69. Guilleminault C, Quo S, Huynh NT, et al. Orthodontic expansion treatment and adenotonsillectomy in the treatment of obstructive sleep apnea in prepubertal children. Sleep 2008;31:953–7.

70. Troulis MJ, Coppe C, O'Neill MJ, et al. Ultrasound: assessment of the distraction osteogenesis wound in patients undergoing mandibular lengthening. J Oral Maxillofac Surg 2003;61:1144–9.

71. Miller JJ, Kahn D, lorenz HP, et al. Infant mandibular distraction with an internal curvilinear device. J Craniofac Surg 2007;18:1403–7.

72. Scolozzi P, Link DW 2nd, Schendel SA. Computer Simulation of curvilinear mandibular distraction: accurancy and predictability. Plast Reconstr Surg 2007;120:1975–80.

73. Schendel SA, Linck DW 3rd. Mandibular distraction osteogenesis by sagittal split asteotomy and intraoral curvilinear distraction. J craniofac Surg 2004;15: 631–5.

74. Paoli JR, Lauwers F, Lacassagne L, et al. Treatment of obstructive sleep apnea syndrome by mandibular elongation using osseous distraction followed by a Le Fort I advancement osteotomy: case report. J Oral Maxillofac Surg 2001;59:216–9.

75. Li KK, Powell NB, Riley RW, et al. Distraction osteogenesis in adult obstructive sleep apnea surgery: a preliminary report. J Oral Maxillofac Surg 2002; 60:6–10.

76. Magliocca K, Helman JI. Distraction osteogenesis in the management of obstructive sleep apnea. In: Bell WH, Guerrero CA, editors. Distraction osteogenesis of the cranifacial skeleton. Hamilton: BC Decker; 2007. p. 431–6.

77. Wang X, Wang XX, Liang C, et al. Distraction osteogenesis in correction of micrognathia accompanying obstructive sleep apnea syndrome. Plast Reconstr Surg 2003;112:1549–57 [discussion: 58–9].

78. Rachmiel A, Aizenbud D, Pillar G, et al. Bilateral mandibular distraction for patients with compromised airway analyzed by three-dimensional CT. Int J Oral Maxillofac Surg 2005;34:9–18.

79. Denny AD, Talisman R, Hanson PR, et al. Mandibular distraction osteogenesis in very young patients

to correct airway obstruction. Plast Reconstr Surg 2001;108:302–11.

80. Castano FJ, Troulis MJ, Glowacki J, et al. Proliferation of masseter myocytes after distraction osteogenesis of the porcine mandible. J Oral Maxillofac Surg 2001;59:302–7.

81. Ilizarov GA. The tension-stress effect on the genesis and growth of tissues. Part I. The influence of stability of fixation and soft-tissue preservation. Clin Orthop Relat Res 1989;249–81.

82. Wang XX, Wang X, Li ZL. Effects of mandibular distraction osteogenesis on the inferior alveolar nerve: an experimental study in monkeys. Plast Reconstr Surg 2002;109:2373–83.

83. Michieli S, Miotti B. Lengthening of mandibular body by gradual surgical-orthodontic distraction. J Oral Surg 1977;35:187–92.

84. Makarov MR, Harper RP, Cope JB, et al. Evaluation of inferior alveolar nerve function during distraction osteogenesis in the dog. J Oral Maxillofac Surg 1998;56:1417–23 [discussion: 24–5].

85. Hu J, Tang Z, Wang D, et al. Changes in the inferior alveolar nerve after mandibular lengthening with different rates of distraction. J Oral Maxillofac Surg 2001;59:1041–5.

86. Bendahan GJ. Distraction osteogenesis versus bilateral sagittal split osteotomy for mandibular advancement [Master of science thesis]. Boston: Harvard University; 2005.

87. Ayoub AF, Duncan CM, McLean GR, et al. Response of patients and families to lengthening of the facial bones by extraoral distraction osteogenesis: a review of 14 patients. Br J Oral Maxillofac Surg 2002;40:397–405.

88. Primrose AC, Broadfoot E, Diner PA, et al. Patients' responses to distraction osteogenesis: a multi-centre study. Int J Oral Maxillofac Surg 2005;34:238–42.

89. Figueroa AA, Polley JW. Clinical controversies in oral and maxillofacial surgery: Part two. External versus internal distraction osteogenesis for the management of severe maxillary hypoplasia: external distraction. J Oral Maxillofac Surg 2008; 66:2598–604.

90. Mofid MM, Manson PN, Robertson BC, et al. Craniofacial distraction osteogenesis: a review of 3278 cases. Plast Reconstr Surg 2001;108: 1103–14 [discussion: 15–7].

91. Ilizarov GA. The tension-stress effect on the genesis and growth of tissues: Part II. The influence of the rate and frequency of distraction. Clin Orthop Relat Res 1989;263–85.

92. Molina F, Ortiz Monasterio F. Mandibular elongation and remodeling by distraction: a farewell to major osteotomies. Plast Reconstr Surg 1995;96:825–40 [discussion: 41–2].

93. Kusnoto B, Figueroa AA, Polley JW. A longitudinal three-dimensional evaluation of the growth pattern in hemifacial microsomia treated by mandibular distraction osteogenesis: a preliminary report. J Craniofac Surg 1999;10:480–6.

94. Ko EW, Hung KF, Huang CS, et al. Correction of facial asymmetry with multiplanar mandible distraction: a one-year follow-up study. Cleft Palate Craniofac J 2004;41:5–12.

95. Klein C, Howaldt HP. Lengthening of the hypoplastic mandible by gradual distraction in childhood: a preliminary report. J Craniomaxillofac Surg 1995;23:68–74.

96. Hollier LH, Kim JH, Grayson B, et al. Mandibular growth after distraction in patients under 48 months of age. Plast Reconstr Surg 1999;103: 1361–70.

97. Carls FR, Sailer HF. Seven years clinical experience with mandibular distraction in children. J Craniomaxillofac Surg 1998;26:197–208.

98. Rachmiel A, Manor R, Peled M, et al. Intraoral distraction osteogenesis of the mandible in hemifacial microsomia. J Oral Maxillofac Surg 2001;59: 728–33.

99. Marquez IM, Fish LC, Stella JP. Two-year follow-up of distraction osteogenesis: its effect on mandibular ramus height in hemifacial microsomia. Am J Orthod Dentofacial Orthop 2000;117:130–9.

100. Huang CS, Ko WC, Lin WY, et al. Mandibular lengthening by distraction osteogenesis in children: a one-year follow-up study. Cleft Palate Craniofac J 1999;36:269–74.

101. van Strijen PJ, Breuning KH, Becking AG, et al. Stability after distraction osteogenesis to lengthen the mandible: results in 50 patients. J Oral Maxillofac Surg 2004;62:304–7.

102. Li KK, Powell NB, Riley RW, et al. Long-term results of maxillomandibular advancement surgery. Sleep Breath 2000;4:137–40.

Index

Note: Page numbers of article titles are in **boldface** type.

A

Acoustic reflection technology, of upper airway in sleep-disordered breathing, 394

Adenoidectomy, for obstructive sleep apnea, 438–439
    adult, 438
    pediatric, 438

Adherence, to CPAP, approaches to improve, 407
    predictors of, 405–406
    prevalence of poor, 405

Aging, role in obstructive sleep apnea, 372

Airflow modeling, steps in, for obstructive sleep apnea syndrome, 395–399
    computer fluid dynamics visualization, 397–399
    generation of numerical meshes, 396–397
    geometry generation with 3-D CT scan, 395–396

Airway, edema after obstructive sleep apnea surgery, 431–432
    obstruction, congenital and infant, distraction osteogenesis for, 464–468
    reconstruction of soft tissues in obstructive sleep apnea, **435–445**
        airway assessment, 437
        anesthetic considerations, 436–437
        base of tongue techniques, 442–443
        epiglottidectomy, 443
        for snoring, 440–442
        Friedman staging, 437
        nasal surgery, 438
        palatopharyngoplasty, 439–440
        structure, 435–436
        tonsillectomy/adenoidectomy in adults and children, 438–438
        tracheotomy, 437

Alcohol, role in obstructive sleep apnea, 373

Analgesia, postoperative, for obstructive sleep apnea surgery, 431

Anatomic factors, in obstructive sleep apnea, 370–371

Anesthetic management, in surgery for obstructive sleep apnea, **425–434**
    for maxillomandibular advancement, 451
    for reconstruction of airway soft tissues in, 436–437
    intraoperative, 427–429
        extubation techniques, 428–429
        intubation techniques, 428

        patient ventilation, 427–428
    postoperative, 429–432
        analgesia, 430
        blood pressure control, 431
        deep vein thrombosis prophylaxis, 431
        discharge criteria, 431
        monitoring, 429
        patient positioning, 429–430
        reducing airway edema, 430–431
        sedatives, 431
        use of CPAP, 430
    preoperative, 426–427
        choice of local, general, or monitored care, 426–427
        communication with anesthesia team, 427
        narcotics and sedative agents, 427
        preoperative medical clearance, 427
        reflux/aspiration precautions, 427
        selection of facility, 426
        use of CPAP, 427

Apnea. *See* Obstructive sleep apnea.

Appliances, oral, for simple snoring, mandibular repositioning, 385
    for snoring and sleep-disordered breathing, **413–420**
        clinical protocol, 415
        compliance and adverse effects, 416–417
        effectiveness compared with CPAP and surgery, 417–418
        overview, 413–415
        prediction of treatment success, 417
        titration protocols, 416

Aspiration precautions, in obstructive sleep apnea surgery, 427

B

Blood pressure control, after obstructive sleep apnea surgery, 432

C

Cephalometric radiography, of upper airway in sleep-disordered breathing, 390–393

Clearance, preoperative medical, for obstructive sleep apnea surgery, 427

Compliance, patient, to CPAP, approaches to improve, 405–407
    with oral appliances for snoring and sleep-disordered breathing, 416–417

doi:10.1016/S1042-3699(09)00101-0
1042-3699/09/$ – see front matter © 2009 Elsevier Inc. All rights reserved.

United States Postal Service
Statement of Ownership, Management, and Circulation
(All Periodicals Publications Except Requester Publications)

1. Publication Title	2. Publication Number	3. Filing Date
Oral and Maxillofacial Surgery Clinics of North America	0 0 6 - 3 6 2	9/15/09

4. Issue Frequency	5. Number of Issues Published Annually	6. Annual Subscription Price
Feb, May, Aug, Nov	4	$271.00

7. Complete Mailing Address of Known Office of Publication (Not printer) (Street, city, county, state, and ZIP+4®)

Elsevier Inc.
360 Park Avenue South
New York, NY 10010-1710

Contact Person
Stephen Bushing
Telephone (Include area code)
215-239-3688

8. Complete Mailing Address of Headquarters or General Business Office of Publisher (Not printer)

Elsevier Inc., 360 Park Avenue South, New York, NY 10010-1710

9. Full Names and Complete Mailing Addresses of Publisher, Editor, and Managing Editor (Do not leave blank)

Publisher (Name and complete mailing address)

John Schrefer, Elsevier, Inc., 1600 John F. Kennedy Blvd. Suite 1800, Philadelphia, PA 19103-2899

Editor (Name and complete mailing address)

John Vassallo, Elsevier, Inc., 1600 John F. Kennedy Blvd. Suite 1800, Philadelphia, PA 19103-2899

Managing Editor (Name and complete mailing address)

Catherine Bewick, Elsevier, Inc., 1600 John F. Kennedy Blvd. Suite 1800, Philadelphia, PA 19103-2899

10. Owner (Do not leave blank. If the publication is owned by a corporation, give the name and address of the corporation immediately followed by the names and addresses of all stockholders owning or holding 1 percent or more of the total amount of stock. If not owned by a corporation, give the names and addresses of the individual owners. If owned by a partnership or other unincorporated firm, give its name and address as well as those of each individual owner. If the publication is published by a nonprofit organization, give its name and address.)

Full Name	Complete Mailing Address
Wholly owned subsidiary of	4520 East-West Highway
Reed/Elsevier, US holdings	Bethesda, MD 20814

11. Known Bondholders, Mortgagees, and Other Security Holders Owning or Holding 1 Percent or More of Total Amount of Bonds, Mortgages, or Other Securities. If none, check box → ☐ None

Full Name	Complete Mailing Address
N/A	

12. Tax Status (For completion by nonprofit organizations authorized to mail at nonprofit rates) (Check one)
The purpose, function, and nonprofit status of this organization and the exempt status for federal income tax purposes:
☐ Has Not Changed During Preceding 12 Months
☐ Has Changed During Preceding 12 Months (Publisher must submit explanation of change with this statement)

PS Form 3526, September 2007 (Page 1 of 3 (Instructions Page 3)) PSN 7530-01-000-9931 PRIVACY NOTICE: See our Privacy policy in www.usps.com

---

13. Publication Title	14. Issue Date for Circulation Data Below
Oral and Maxillofacial Surgery Clinics of North America	August 2009

15. Extent and Nature of Circulation		Average No. Copies Each Issue During Preceding 12 Months	No. Copies of Single Issue Published Nearest to Filing Date
a. Total Number of Copies (Net press run)		2762	2648
b. Paid Circulation (By Mail and Outside the Mail)	(1) Mailed Outside-County Paid Subscriptions Stated on PS Form 3541. (Include paid distribution above nominal rate, advertiser's proof copies, and exchange copies)	1753	1680
	(2) Mailed In-County Paid Subscriptions Stated on PS Form 3541 (Include paid distribution above nominal rate, advertiser's proof copies, and exchange copies)		
	(3) Paid Distribution Outside the Mails Including Sales Through Dealers and Carriers, Street Vendors, Counter Sales, and Other Paid Distribution Outside USPS®	294	301
	(4) Paid Distribution by Other Classes Mailed Through the USPS (e.g. First-Class Mail®)		
c. Total Paid Distribution (Sum of 15b (1), (2), (3), and (4))	►	2047	1981
d. Free or Nominal Rate Distribution (By Mail and Outside the Mail)	(1) Free or Nominal Rate Outside-County Copies Included on PS Form 3541	190	201
	(2) Free or Nominal Rate In-County Copies Included on PS Form 3541		
	(3) Free or Nominal Rate Copies Mailed at Other Classes Through the USPS (e.g. First-Class Mail)		
	(4) Free or Nominal Rate Distribution Outside the Mail (Carriers or other means)		
e. Total Free or Nominal Rate Distribution (Sum of 15d (1), (2), (3) and (4))	►	190	201
f. Total Distribution (Sum of 15c and 15e)	►	2237	2182
g. Copies not Distributed (See instructions to publishers #4 (page #3))	►	525	466
h. Total (Sum of 15f and g)	►	2762	2648
i. Percent Paid (15c divided by 15f times 100)		91.51%	90.79%

16. Publication of Statement of Ownership

☐ If the publication is a general publication, publication of this statement is required. Will be printed in the November 2009 issue of this publication. ☐ Publication not required

17. Signature and Title of Editor, Publisher, Business Manager, or Owner

Stephen R. Bushing — Subscription Services Coordinator

Date: September 15, 2009

Stephen R. Bushing – Subscription Services Coordinator

I certify that all information furnished on this form is true and complete. I understand that anyone who furnishes false or misleading information on this form or who omits material or information requested on the form may be subject to criminal sanctions (including fines and imprisonment) and/or civil sanctions (including civil penalties).

PS Form 3526, September 2007 (Page 2 of 3)

Moving?

Make sure your subscription moves with you!

To notify us of your new address, find your **Clinics Account Number** (located on your mailing label above your name), and contact customer service at:

Email: journalscustomerservice-usa@elsevier.com

800-654-2452 (subscribers in the U.S. & Canada)
314-447-8871 (subscribers outside of the U.S. & Canada)

Fax number: 314-447-8029

Elsevier Health Sciences Division
Subscription Customer Service
3251 Riverport Lane
Maryland Heights, MO 63043

ELSEVIER

Printed and bound by CPI Group (UK) Ltd, Croydon, CR0 4YY

03/10/2024

01040352-0013